Chest X-Ray
Interpretation

pocket tutor

Chest X-Ray Interpretation

pocket tutor

Mike Darby BA MRCP FRCR
Consultant Radiologist
North Bristol NHS Trust
Bristol, UK

Anthony Edey MRCP FRCR
Consultant Radiologist
North Bristol NHS Trust
Bristol, UK

Ladli Chandratreya MBBS DMRD FRCR
Consultant Radiologist
North Bristol NHS Trust
Bristol, UK

Nick Maskell FRCP DM
Senior Lecturer and Respiratory Consultant
University of Bristol
Bristol, UK

JP
medical
publishers

Published by JP Medical Ltd, 83 Victoria Street, London, SW1H 0HW, UK

Tel: +44 (0)20 3170 8910 Fax: +44 (0)20 3008 6180

Email: info@jpmedpub.com Web: www.jpmedpub.com

ISBN: 978-1-907816-06-2

British Library Cataloguing in Publication Data
A catalogue record for this book is available from the British Library

Library of Congress Cataloging in Publication Data
A catalog record for this book is available from the Library of Congress

JP Medical Ltd is a subsidiary of Jaypee Brothers Medical Publishers (P) Ltd, New Delhi, India

Publisher:	Richard Furn
Development Editor:	Paul Mayhew
Editorial Assistant:	Katrina Rimmer
Design:	Designers Collective Ltd
Indexing:	Indexing Specialists (UK) Ltd

Typeset, printed and bound in India.

Preface

We have written *Pocket Tutor Chest X-Ray Interpretation* in a concise fashion to help the reader develop a good basic understanding of how to interpret the chest radiograph. A step-by-step approach is essential to this, and so this book presents a systematic method in order to avoid mistakes. It also highlights a number of pitfalls to watch out for when interpreting chest radiographs.

The opening chapter explains the basic concepts of chest radiology, including some elementary physics. Chapters two and three then present the building blocks for understanding normal and abnormal chest radiology, respectively. The remaining chapters concisely describe common clinical disorders for which chest radiology is an important investigative tool. These include brief clinical scenarios together with labelled chest X-rays to inform the reader. Another key feature of the book is the *Clinical Insight and Guiding Principle* boxes which draw upon our collective personal experience.

This book is not exhaustive, but we hope that it is comprehensive in covering the main conditions that can affect the chest radiograph. We hope you will enjoy reading it, that it will serve as a handy companion for quick reference and that the knowledge you gain will help guide you in the management of your patients.

Mike Darby
Anthony Edey
Ladli Chandratreya
Nick Maskell
February 2012

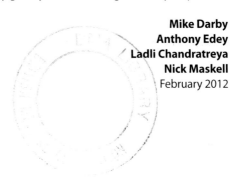

Contents

First principles

1.1 Physics of X-rays

X-rays are a type of electromagnetic radiation with wavelengths between 0.01 and 10 nm. On the electromagnetic spectrum, the wavelength of X-rays is shorter than that of ultraviolet radiation and longer than that of gamma radiation. Shorter wavelength X-rays (0.10–0.01 nm) are referred to as 'hard' because they can penetrate solid objects. It is these that are used in medical imaging. Since their discovery in 1895 by the German physicist Wilhelm Roentgen, X-rays have been used widely for medical imaging and remain key to diagnosing and treating patients.

X-ray production

X-rays are produced in an X-ray tube (**Figure 1.1**) by firing electrons at about half the speed of light from the cathode towards a metal target, the anode. The target is usually made from an alloy of tungsten. On impact with the target, the kinetic energy of the electrons is converted into X-rays (1%) and heat (99%). The target deflects and focuses the X-rays to form a beam.

X-ray attenuation

The X-ray beam is directed at the patient in a short pulse and is absorbed (attenuated) by the tissues of the body. Materials with a high electron density, such as bone, attenuate the beam to a greater extent than soft tissue, water or air. Therefore the beam

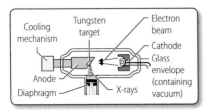

Figure 1.1 An X-ray tube. Electrons are emitted by a cathode into the vacuum, emitting X-rays when hitting the anode at the right (i.e. current) speed.

that emerges from the patient carries a pattern of intensity that reflects the physical anatomy through which it has passed.

Image production

The beam that emerges is directed onto either a photostimulated phosphor plate or a flat panel detector. These methods of image capture have superseded photographic film and allow rapid production of digital images.

Radiation risks and use

The risk to the patient from a chest X-ray is minimal. However, all health care professionals who request X-rays should be familiar with and keep in mind the potential dangers of radiation.

When X-rays are absorbed by tissue, they cause chemical, molecular and subsequently biological damage (in a timespan of seconds, minutes and decades, respectively). The direct consequences of radiation to the patient are categorised as deterministic or stochastic. Deterministic effects (e.g. skin damage, cataracts and sterility) are relevant to radiotherapy, and to a lesser extent interventional radiology, and occur once a threshold dose of radiation is administered. Stochastic effects (e.g. cancers) are relevant to diagnostic radiology and reflect the probability of harm, which is assumed to be proportional to dose (measured in mSv). Data to support estimates of radiation risk have been derived mostly from follow-up of survivors of the 1945 atomic bombing of Hiroshima and Nagasaki. The following facts help put the risks of chest X-rays in context.

- Background exposure to radiation for the whole population is 2.5 mSv/year.
- A 7-h airline flight exposes passengers to 0.02 mSv.
- The overall lifetime risk of cancer for the general population is about 40%.
- A chest X-ray has a dose of 0.1 mSv and increases a patient's lifetime risk of cancer by about 0.001%.

Use of radiation in medical practice is governed in the UK by the Ionising Radiation (Medical Exposure) Regulations 2000. These lay down the basic measures to protect persons from the dangers of medical radiation exposure. Legal responsibility for protecting those exposed to medical radiation lies with the person administering ionising radiation.

1.2 Positioning the patient and obtaining the image

Several techniques are used to visualise the structures of the thorax, but the chest X-ray remains the most common radiological examination. The difference in densities and resulting contrast between structures of the thorax make good visualisation and assessment of the lungs possible. This section deals with various techniques in plain chest radiography regarding patient positioning and obtaining the image.

Frontal chest X-ray

A frontal view of the chest is always obtained when a plain chest X-ray is requested. It is most often a posteroanterior (PA) view. Alternatively, an anteroposterior (AP) view is used if the patient is unable to stand or sit for a PA view. Lateral, apical, lordotic and decubitus views are occasionally obtained as adjuncts to the frontal (PA or AP) X-ray.

Posteroanterior X-rays

The PA view is obtained by positioning the patient facing the film cassette, with the shoulders rotated forwards to project the scapulae away from the lungs. With the chin raised, the chest and shoulders are in contact with the cassette. The view is centred on the midline at the level of the 5th thoracic vertebra and exposure obtained in arrested full inspiration (**Figure 1.2**). The following allow a PA film to be interpreted confidently.
- Sternal ends of the clavicles equidistant from the vertebral spinous process.
- Clavicles not obscuring the lung apices (**Figure 1.2a**).
- Lungs well inflated, allowing 10 posterior ribs to be seen above the diaphragm on each side (**Figure 1.2a**).
- Between 2.5 and 5 cm of lung fields visible above the clavicles
- Lateral borders of the ribs equidistant from the vertebral column.

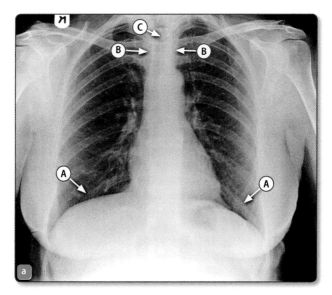

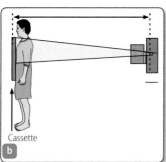

Figure 1.2 (a) Posteroanterior (PA) chest X-ray in good inspiration with posterior tenth ribs **A** visualised. Medial ends of clavicles **B** equidistant from vertebral spinous process **C**. (b) Positioning of the patient in a PA view, with the patient facing the cassette. The X-ray beam is behind the patient, centred on the 5th thoracic vertebra.

- Superior thoracic vertebrae visible through the heart.
- Well-defined costophrenic angles and margins of the mediastinum, heart and diaphragm.

Posteroanterior X-ray in expiration The PA X-ray in expiration is obtained to better visualise a small apical pneumothorax or to show the effects of an obstructing inhaled foreign body (i.e. air trapping). All other positioning factors remain the same as for an inspiratory PA X-ray.

Anteroposterior X-rays

The AP view (**Figure 1.3**) is used as an alternative to a PA view in patients who are very ill or unable to comply with the positioning requirements of a PA view. The AP view is occasionally used as an adjunct to further assess an opacity seen on a PA view.

Anteroposterior X-rays appear different from PA X-rays in multiple ways.
- The scapulae may obscure the lungs (**Figure 1.3a**), because AP X-rays are usually obtained in patients who are unable to project their shoulders downwards and forwards.
- The AP view magnifies the heart, because it is further away from the cassette compared with in a PA view, making assessment of cardiac enlargement difficult (**Figure 1.3a**).
- The clavicles are projected higher than in a PA view (**Figure 1.3a**).

Anteroposterior erect X-ray

The AP erect view is obtained with the patient standing or sitting with the back against the cassette and the upper edge of the cassette above the apex of the lungs. The ray is directed horizontally and centred on the suprasternal notch (**Figure 1.3b**).

Lateral chest X-ray

A lateral view of the chest is no longer routinely obtained. It is instead sometimes used as an additional view for localising a mass lesion (**Figure 1.4a**) or confirming a hiatus hernia if further assessment by computerised tomography is not possible.

The patient is positioned with the side of interest in contact with the cassette and the sagittal plane parallel to it (**Figure 1.4b**). The arms are raised above the head. The horizontal ray is centred

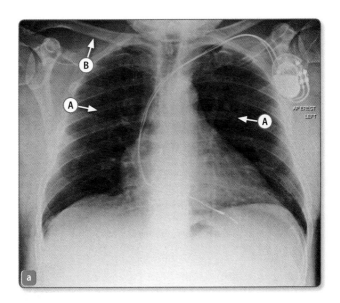

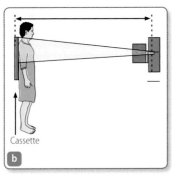

Figure 1.3 (a) Anteroposterior (AP) chest X-ray with the scapulae overlapping more of the lung fields. The heart appears larger on an AP view. (A) Medial margins of scapulae. (B) Clavicles projected above the lung apices. (b) Positioning of the patient for an AP view. The patient faces the X-ray beam with the back against the cassette.

on the midaxillary line. Infirm and very ill patients are unable to comply with this positioning.

The sternum and vertebral column are better visualised on a lateral view (**Figure 1.5**). The lateral view can also often better show lesions obscured on the PA view (e.g. lobar

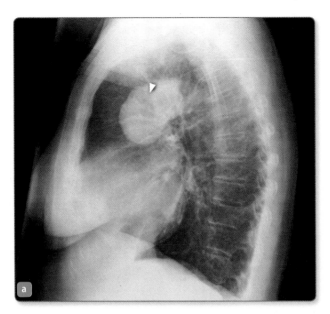

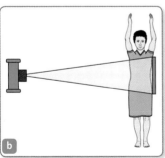

Figure 1.4 (a) Lateral chest X-ray showing a mass (arrowhead) next to the hilum. The mass is better localised with an additional posteroanterior view (Figure 1.5a). (b) Positioning of the patient for a lateral view. The patient has one side in contact with the cassette, while the X-ray beam is centred on the midaxillary line of the opposite side.

atelectasis, posterior recess lesions, fluid in fissures and anterior mediastinal masses). Conversely, lesions seen clearly on a PA view can be obscured by the mediastinum or overlapping lung fields. A lateral view involves a much higher radiation dose than a PA view.

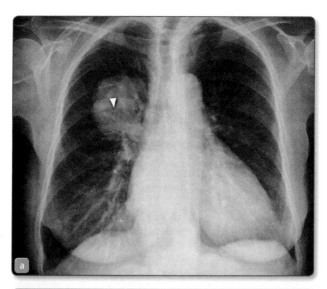

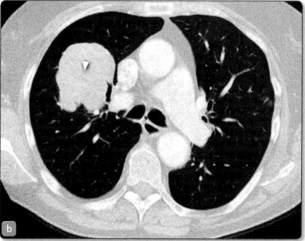

Figure 1.5 (a) Posteroanterior chest X-ray showing a mass in the right upper zone (arrowhead) (same patient as in Figure 1.4). (b) Computerised tomography scan confirming the position of the mass (arrowhead).

Other views of the chest

Additional views can be helpful, including:
- decubitus views, which show air–fluid levels and can show subpulmonic effusions that are not loculated
- supine views, which are obtained for very ill and debilitated patients, for babies and, rarely, for subpulmonic effusions.

Three other views are used less frequently:
- apical and lordotic views to better visualise the apices and middle lobe atelectasis, respectively (now rarely used)
- oblique views, no longer routinely used to show rib fractures.

1.3 Radiographic densities

The principle of imaging using X-rays is to differentiate body parts through differences in their constituents. Body tissues vary in density and therefore the amount of radiation they absorb.

The densest abnormalities visible on an X-ray are metallic and appear white. They include inhaled or swallowed foreign bodies or surgical artefacts (e.g. pacemakers).

Bone and calcific lesions (e.g. calcified nodules from previous tuberculosis) have the highest density of the body tissues of the chest. They will absorb most radiation and therefore appear whiter than surrounding tissue.

The soft tissues (e.g. body wall, heart and abdominal organs) are similar in density so appear mid-grey. Layers of fat in the chest wall may appear slightly darker.

Air has the lowest density and appears black. Lungs contain mostly air and are therefore grey or black.

Nodule assessment depends on the ability to identify the higher density of the nodules compared with surrounding soft tissue. Calcified nodules resulting from previous tuberculosis or chickenpox pneumonia (**Figure 1.6**) are benign.

The silhouette sign

The edges of structures such as the heart, diaphragm and masses are visible only if a difference in density exists between them and the adjacent tissue. This is the silhouette sign. It is

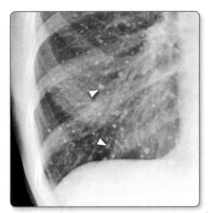

Figure 1.6 Chest X-ray showing calcified lung nodules caused by old chickenpox pneumonia. Multiple nodules (arrowheads) have a whiteness or density similar to or greater than that of bone. They are calcific and therefore almost certainly benign.

helpful because if an edge of a structure that is usually visible is no longer visible, it means that the adjacent lung is of the same density, i.e. more solid than usual (**Figure 1.7**).

Most lung diseases increase density, e.g. pneumonia or tumour fills air spaces with material. Lower density (darker) pathological changes such as a pneumothorax or emphysematous bullae are seen when there is increased air in the region.

Description of abnormalities

The cause of abnormalities seen on a chest X-ray is not always immediately apparent. Using descriptions such as size, density and clarity of margins helps to categorise lesions, and making a diagnosis becomes easier when these findings are put together. Thus the interpretation of X-rays is similar to a clinical examination; a diagnosis is more likely when all the signs are considered together rather than when a single aspect is focused on. For example, if an opacity is described as an ill-defined area of shadowing without discrete edges and with an air bronchogram, it is almost certainly infective consolidation. However, if it is a well-defined opacity with clear margins, it is most likely a tumour.

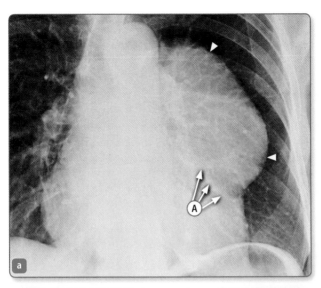

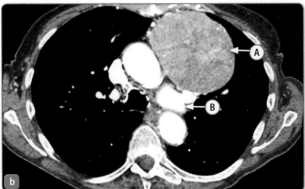

Figure 1.7 Mediastinal mass causing loss of normal silhouette. (a) Chest X-ray. The edge of the mass is clear because of the sharp demarcation with the adjacent lung (arrowheads). (A) The left heart border is obscured by a large mediastinal mass (thymoma) lying next to it; with no difference in density, the structures appear continuous. (b) Computed tomography scan. (A) The left border of the radiographic opacity is created by the lateral aspect of the mass. (B) Normal hilar structures are outlined by the aerated lung and so are visible on the chest X-ray.

1.4 Picture archiving and communication systems: image optimisation and pitfalls

In most countries, a picture archiving and communication system (PACS) is used to deliver imaging to clinicians. With previous film-based systems, images were made singly and the image could not be manipulated once produced.

Picture archiving and communication systems allow easy electronic storage with instant simultaneous access at many distant sites. The PACS may be integrated with other patient data and interface with patient medical records. Reports can be made available electronically without the need to post paper copies. The images can also be manipulated to improve analysis.

Disadvantages of picture archiving and communication systems

It has always been necessary to view X-rays in good viewing conditions because excess background light impairs visualisation, hence the darkening of radiologists' viewing rooms. This is even more important with PACS workstations. An old-fashioned light box emits much more light than a computer screen, so if a monitor is used any outside glare from lights or the sun will decrease visibility. If films are viewed in wards, it is essential to move monitors away from direct sunlight and ward lights, preferably into a side room.

Advantages of PACS systems

Radiologists usually have expensive high-quality screens in specialised viewing rooms. Therefore review images that are insufficiently clear with a radiologist in the radiology department.

Radiology systems have many software manipulations to facilitate image assessment, but many of these will also be available on the ward or clinic-based computers.

- Window level (i.e. contrast and brightness): adjusting the whiteness and contrast makes some areas more visible, but take care to avoid losing detail elsewhere.

- Magnification: magnifying part of an image may help characterise its nature (**Figure 1.8**).

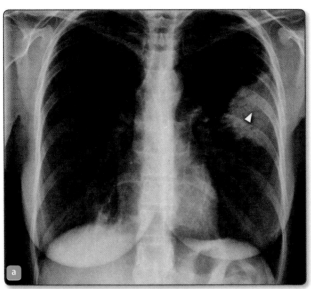

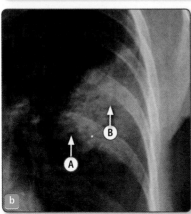

Figure 1.8 Magnification.
(a) Chest X-ray showing a large opacity (arrowhead) in the left upper zone.
(b) Detail can be improved by magnifying part of the image. Ill-defined edges (A) suggest consolidation. Branching lucencies in the lesion (B) are now visible, consistent with consolidation (air bronchogram).

- Size measurements: many measuring tools are available on PACS software, most commonly for measuring sizes (e.g. of the heart in **Figure 1.9**).

1.5 Errors of perception and interpretation

Image analysis and interpretation is a complex multistep process with anatomical, physiological, neuropsychological and psychoemotional components. Errors are therefore common and interpretation of chest X-rays is notoriously difficult, with false negative rates of 20–30% and false positive rates of 2–5%.

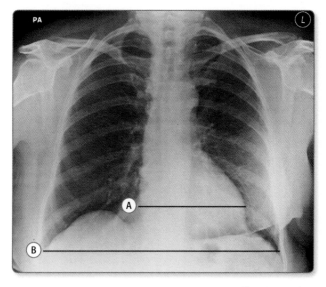

Figure 1.9 Measurements. Chest X-ray showing cardiac size Ⓐ (15.5 cm) and thoracic diameter Ⓑ (34 cm). The cardiothoracic ratio is 15.5:34.0, meaning that the heart size is normal. Incidentally, in this case there has been a left mastectomy and breast implant: the breast border is asymmetrical and the soft tissues overlying the left breast area are of increased density.

The mechanics of vision

The eye is better suited to daytime hunting and identifying predators than to detecting small pulmonary nodules. Only the fovea, which measures 1.5 mm across, contains cones, the receptors used to analyse fine detail. To compensate for this small population of cones, the eye executes rapid jerky movements (saccades) to maximise exposure of the fovea to the scene it is surveying. However, during motion the fovea is blind, acquiring data only at rest. Therefore vision is a non-continuous process with noise and image blur during movement interspersed with high-resolution static vision.

Lesion identification

Identification of lesions relies on the abnormality lying in the field of active search, its physical characteristics and recognition that it is abnormal. Therefore the first step towards reducing misses is to follow a systematic pattern of review (see section 2.4). The size, density, contour and location of a lesion all affect the ability to recognise its presence; a small fatty lesion lying behind the heart will probably be undetected.

Recognition of the abnormal requires familiarity with the normal and comes only with practice. Until you have seen thousands of chest X-rays, it is worth asking a senior colleague or a radiologist for help when you feel unsure.

Cognitive errors

Cognitive errors are essentially human errors and come in many guises. Understanding the nature of these errors will help you to reduce them; some examples follow.

- **Satisfaction of search:** having spotted an error, you stop looking and miss further potentially more significant findings.
- **Availability bias:** having recently seen a patient with, or more importantly missed the diagnosis of, a particular disease, you assume that the next patient has the same disease. Conversely, if you have not seen a particular disease for a long time you will not think about it for the current patient.

- **Capture:** you get interrupted in the middle of systematically reviewing a patient's chest X-ray and do not complete your analysis; you may thereby miss a pneumothorax.
- **Gambler's fallacy:** having recently seen several patients with the same problem, you assume that the next patient cannot have the same diagnosis. The same assumption is made by gamblers, who after flipping heads on a coin 10 times in a row falsely assume that the likelihood of heads again is lower than before.

Guiding principle

Minimise errors as follows.

- Give your eyes a chance: view images on the best screen you can find, ideally in a dimly lit room; there is a reason radiologists sit in the dark!
- Confirm that you are looking at the correct patient's X-rays
- Develop a systematic approach to interpreting chest X-rays
- Avoid interruptions
- Have an open mind and decide on the radiological signs and patterns before considering diagnoses
- When in doubt, seek help

- **Anchoring:** you form an opinion early in the analytic process and then seek evidence to support your diagnosis, prematurely discarding contrary evidence. The first diagnosis gains its own momentum, making consideration of an alternative diagnosis more difficult.
- **Alliterative errors:** previous reports or opinions from others, which may be incorrect, influence your thinking, making it more difficult for you to think of other possible diagnoses.
- **Overconfidence:** the tendency to believe that you know more than you do!

Understanding the normal chest X-ray

2.1 Normal chest anatomy

Normal views

Posteroanterior chest X-ray

The frontal posteroanterior (PA) chest X-ray is a fundamental part of a respiratory examination. It gives a very low radiation dose. Also, because of the greater differences in tissue densities than in, for example, an abdominal X-ray, it shows small lesions and fine detail well. Computerised tomography (CT) scans show detail much better but give a radiation dose 3–400 times greater, are much less readily available and are considerably more expensive.

To assess abnormalities on a chest X-ray, it is essential to understand the basic anatomy of the chest and the normal positions and appearances of the visible structures. Key anatomical structures to identify on a PA radiograph are shown in **Figure 2.1**.

Lateral chest X-ray

The lateral chest X-ray (**Figure 2.2**) is generally less useful than the frontal view because the two lungs are superimposed and the anatomy of the two sides is non-identical. However, a lateral view shows some of the hidden areas of the lungs. For example, the posterior costophrenic recesses lie behind the diaphragm and much of the left lower lobe can be hidden behind the heart. A lateral view also helps localise items to specific lobes.

Clinical insight

A lateral chest X-ray is useful to confirm a lesion is in the lung, and to localise which lobe it is in

Assessing normal anatomy

Airways and fissures

Airways and fissures are useful landmarks for assessing lung and mediastinal anatomy. Observation of finer detail is sometimes difficult (e.g. if a patient is very large or if the film

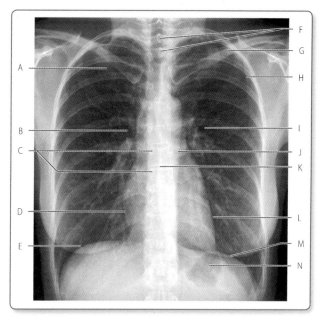

Figure 2.1 PA chest X-ray showing normal anatomy. Ⓐ Anterior end of the right first rib. Count down from here to assess expansion of the chest. The diaphragm is crossed by the 5th to 7th ribs. Ⓑ Right hilar point, formed by the meeting of the horizontal fissure and vessels from the upper and lower zones. Ⓒ Pedicles of thoracic spine. Ⓓ Right heart border, formed mainly from the border of the right atrium. Ⓔ Dome of the right hemidiaphragm, crossed by the anterior end of the right 6th rib. Ⓕ Spinous processes of the thoracic spine seen through the lucency of the trachea. Ⓖ Left clavicle. Ⓗ Border of the left scapula. Ⓘ Left hilar point, slightly higher than the right and formed by the crossing of vessels from the upper and lower zones. Ⓙ Edge of descending thoracic aorta. Ⓚ Disc space of thoracic spine, which should be just visible on well-exposed film. Ⓛ Left heart border, formed by the edge of the left and right ventricles. Ⓜ Dome of the left hemidiaphragm, usually slightly lower than the right. Ⓝ Gas in stomach lumen.

is suboptimal in a very ill patient), but it can help differentiate normal from abnormal. Enlargements of parts of the film, sometimes with additional alteration of contrast and density, may make some structures more visible (**Figures 2.3 and 2.4**).

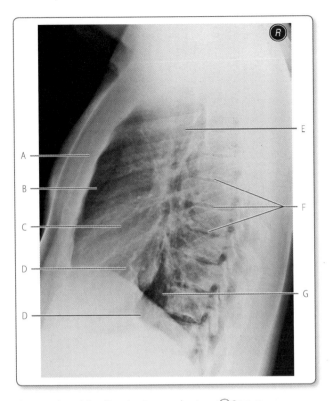

Figure 2.2 Lateral chest X-ray showing normal anatomy. (A) Sternum.
(B) Retrosternal space, hidden on a posteroanterior (PA) chest X-ray. (C) Heart.
(D) Right and left hemidiaphragms. The stomach is below the left hemidiaphragm,
which merges with the heart border. The right hemidiaphragm is usually higher than
the left. (E) Lucency of the trachea. (F) Intervertebral thoracic disc spaces. The spine
should appear gradually more lucent from the top down to the bottom because less
soft tissue overlies the lower parts. (G) Retrocardiac space, hidden on a PA chest X-ray.

Mediastinal features Note the following when assessing the
mediastinum.

- If the film is correctly centred, the upper spinous processes
  are projected over the middle of the trachea. The trachea

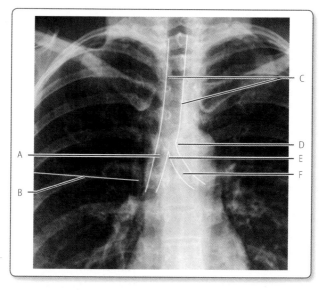

Figure 2.3 AP chest X-ray with superimposed outlines of fissures and airways.
(A) Right main bronchus. (B) Position of major (horizontal) fissure. (C) Lateral
borders of the trachea. (D) Indentation on the trachea from the aortic knuckle.
(E) Carina. (F) Left main bronchus.

and main bronchi have incomplete rings of cartilage, which
frequently calcify with increasing age.

- A left-sided aorta deviates the lower trachea to the right. The
  left lateral border of the descending aorta is visible alongside
  the spine.
- The left main bronchus is more horizontal and longer than
  the right, with the left main pulmonary artery passing over it.
- The hilar points are where the upper and lower zone lung
  vascular structures cross medially. The horizontal fissure,
  if seen, should reach the right hilar point. The left hilum is
  slightly higher than the right.

The fissures   The fissures are seen only in a minority of cases and
may appear discontinuous. All three may be visible on a lateral

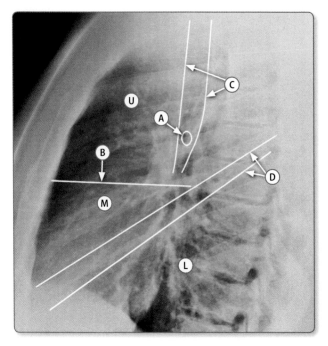

Figure 2.4 AP chest X-ray with superimposed outlines of fissures and airways.
Ⓐ Position of carina. The left main bronchus is seen end on because it passes horizontally. Ⓑ Position of horizontal (major) fissure. Ⓒ Borders of trachea. Ⓓ Positions of right and left oblique (minor) fissures. Ⓤ Upper lobes. Ⓜ Middle lobe and lingula. Ⓛ Lower lobes.

film. However, on a frontal X-ray only the horizontal fissure is usually seen because the edges of the oblique fissures are usually not visible unless they are rotated.

The upper and lower lobes overlap considerably because the minor fissures pass obliquely backwards and upwards. Therefore on the frontal X-ray a lesion in the midzone could be in either lobe, and a lateral view is useful to show which one. The right lung has three lobes with separate arterial and airway supply. The left has only two. On this side, the lingula occupies the region of the right middle lobe but is actually part of the upper lobe.

Lung parenchyma The pulmonary vasculature is a combination of veins, arteries and airways. The structures should have a branching pattern that tapers towards the periphery. Few, if any, markings should be visible in the peripheral subpleural centimetre of lung.

Visualisation of edges The mediastinal and diaphragmatic edges are seen only if aerated lung is next to them. Knowledge of lobar anatomy will help in identifying the position of opacities, because the edge effect is lost if a soft tissue density lesion abuts a structure. Therefore if the right heart border is not visible, the abnormality is in the middle lobe; and if the left heart border is not visible, the lingular lobe. If one side of the diaphragm is not visible, then the pathological change lies in one of the lower lobes.

The normal diaphragm

The diaphragm consists of a large central tendon that is dome-shaped and connects with a sheet of thin muscle to the xiphisternum and 7th to 12th ribs. Bands of crura also connect the diaphragm to the upper three lumbar vertebrae as slings enclosing the main openings, through which pass the aorta and oesophagus.

The position of the diaphragm is best assessed on a PA chest X-ray (**Figure 2.5**) by counting which of the anterior ribs crosses the midpoint. The right should lie between the 5th and 7th ribs; the left is slightly lower by up to 2.5 cm.

A diaphragm lower than the 7th rib usually signifies hyperinflated lungs, as seen in asthma or chronic obstructive pulmonary disease. However, it can be normal in young healthy adults who are able to take a particularly good inspiration.
A high diaphragm can suggest the following:
- poor inspiration (e.g. postoperatively or because of severe pain)
- pulmonary fibrosis causing shrinking lungs
- atelectasis of part of the lung

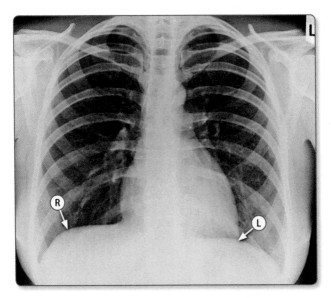

Figure 2.5 Chest X-ray showing the normal position of the diaphragm. (R) Right hemidiaphragm crossed by the anterior 6th rib. (L) Left hemidiaphragm, slightly lower than the right.

2.2 Normal variants

Azygos lobe or fissure

The azygos is the most commonly seen accessory fissure on X-ray. It occurs in 1% of the population and is not associated with any increase in disease susceptibility. It occurs because of abnormal migration of the azygos vein during development. The vein usually migrates from the chest wall to lie in the right tracheobronchial angle, where it joins the superior vena cava. If migration is incomplete, it carries layers of visceral and parietal pleura through the upper lobe to cause an apparent fissure (**Figure 2.6**).

The azygos lobe is not a true lobe. It is a part of the upper lobe, with a normal pattern of bronchovascular anatomy.

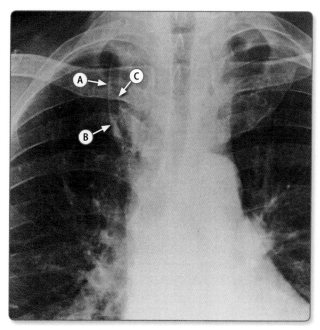

Figure 2.6 Chest X-ray showing azygos lobe demarcated by the azygos fissure Ⓐ containing the azygos vein Ⓑ in its lower part. Ⓒ The azygos lobe.

Accessory or incomplete fissures

Other accessory fissures are commonly seen on CT and are occasionally apparent on X-ray. They must lie tangential to the X-ray beam to be visible, and appear as thin, straight, linear opacities. The inferior accessory fissure separates the medial basal segment of the lower lobe and is more common on the right.

Right-sided aorta

A right-sided aortic arch (**Figure 2.7**) is present in about 0.1% of the population and in adults is rarely associated with other, usually cardiac, abnormalities. It mimics a right superior

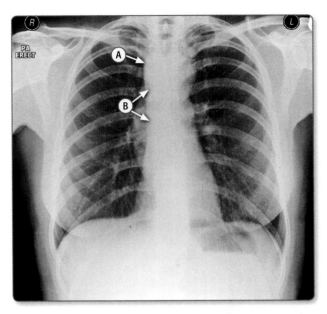

Figure 2.7 Chest X-ray showing right-sided aortic arch. (A) Right-sided aortic knuckle indenting the lower right trachea. (B) Descending aortic margin crossing to the left in a posterior mediastinum.

mediastinal mass, but the diagnosis should be evident if it indents the lower right trachea (**Figure 2.7**) and the usual left aortic knuckle is absent. CT will make the diagnosis clear if doubt exists.

Dextrocardia

Dextrocardia (**Figure 2.8**) is rare. It may be associated with mirror imaging reversal of all chest and abdominal contents (situs inversus totalis). It is more commonly isolated and the aortic arch usually left-sided.

Clinical insight

Rarer aortic anomalies (e.g. double aortic arch) may present earlier with tracheal or oesophageal obstruction. Mirror image reversal of arch and branches is strongly associated with cyanotic congenital heart disease.

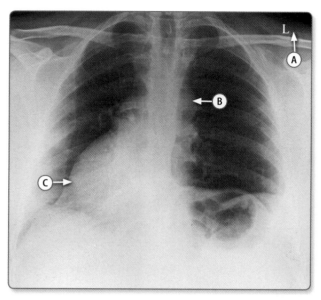

Figure 2.8 Chest X-ray showing dextrocardia. (A) Side marker. (B) Left-sided aortic knuckle. (C) Cardiac apex pointing to the right.

Clinical insight

When in situs inversus form, dextrocardia may be associated with other abnormalities. For example, complications of Kartagener syndrome (ciliary dyskinesia syndrome) include bronchiectasis, sinusitis, otitis and infertility.

Clinical insight

Ossified or non-ossified cervical ribs may cause symptoms if they compress the brachial plexus or subclavian vessels.

Rib anomalies

Ribs may be congenitally bifid (**Figure 2.9**), fused (**Figure 2.10**) or hypoplastic. The 3rd and 4th ribs are the ribs most commonly fused or bifid. They are almost always asymptomatic but may be mistaken for a pulmonary mass. The 1st rib is the one most likely to appear small.

Cervical ribs (**Figure 2.11**) originate from the 7th cervical vertebra and may be confused

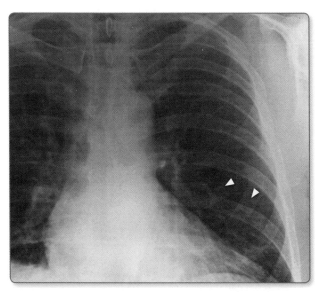

Figure 2.9 Chest X-ray showing congenital anomalies of ribs. The left 4th rib is bifid (arrowheads).

with hypoplastic 1st ribs. Cervical spine X-rays may be needed to confirm the vertebra of origin. Non-ossified cervical ribs may not be apparent on X-ray.

Diaphragm variants

Normal variants of diaphragm contour occur that are usually asymptomatic. Examples include hernias and eventrations.

Bochdalek hernia

A Bochdalek hernia usually contains abdominal fat but can appear mass-like on a chest X-ray (**Figure 2.12a**). It lies posteriorly and medially, more commonly on the left. The hernia results from a small weakness of the diaphragm and can vary with inspiration. A lateral X-ray or comparison with old films may help to make the diagnosis, but CT should be done if doubt exists (**Figure 2.12b**).

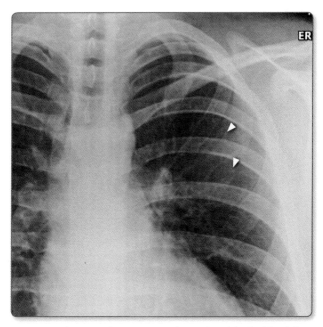

Figure 2.10 Chest X-ray showing congenital anomalies of ribs. The left 3rd rib is bifid and fused (arrowheads).

Eventration of the diaphragm

Eventration of the diaphragm is an anterior bulge of the diaphragm caused by the muscular component being replaced by a thin tendinous sheet. It is usually asymptomatic unless extensive.

Partial eventration is more common on the right and is seen as an anterior, medial, smooth hump of the diaphragm (**Figure 2.13**). It is usually a third to a half of the total surface. A lateral X-ray should confirm the cause (**Figure 2.14**).

Complete eventration is more frequent on the left. It appears and acts more like a paralysed hemidiaphragm because the muscular portion is totally deficient.

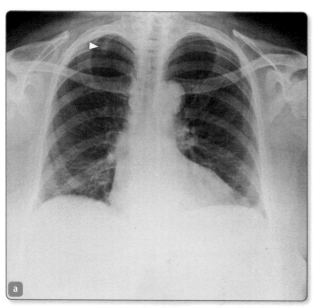

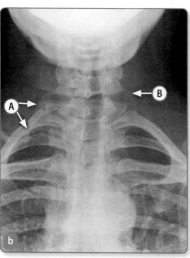

Figure 2.11 Chest X-ray and cervical spine X-ray. (a) Right cervical rib (arrowhead). (b) Cervical spine X-ray shows Ⓐ the right cervical rib more clearly, and normal appearance of the left transverse process of Ⓑ the 7th cervical vertebra.

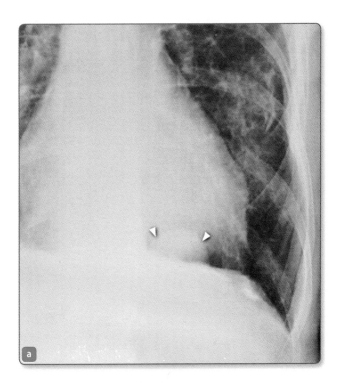

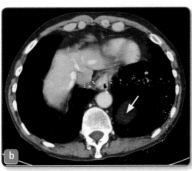

Figure 2.12 Chest X-ray showing Bochdalek hernia. (a) Hump (arrowhead) next to medial border of diaphragm. (b) Computerised tomography scan of the lung base, showing the mass (arrowhead) to be fat continuous with the subdiaphragmatic contents.

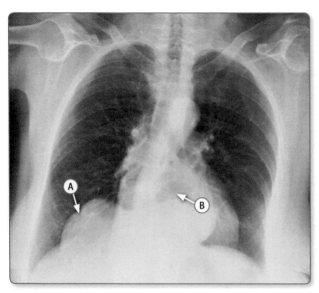

Figure 2.13 PA chest X-ray showing eventration of the right hemidiaphragm. Of incidental note is a large hiatus hernia. (A) Bulge of anterior right diaphragm. (B) Air–fluid level in the hernia.

2.3 Artefacts

Nipple shadows

Nipples may be visible as small nodular opacities in the lower chest (**Figure 2.15a**). They may be confused with intrapulmonary nodules.

Skin folds and skin lesions

Skin folds may sometimes mimic pathological changes. They are visible when

Clinical insight

Never assume that apparent nodules are nipple shadows. Always confirm by a repeat X-ray with nipple markers (**Figure 2.15b**).

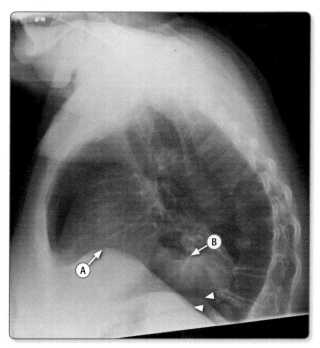

Figure 2.14 Lateral chest X-ray showing eventration of the right hemidiaphragm (same patient as in Figure 2.13). Ⓐ Bulge of anterior right diaphragm. Ⓑ Air–fluid level in the hernia. Normal posterior positions of both posterior hemidiaphragms (arrowheads).

there is an abrupt transition of density between the soft tissue of skin and adjacent air. They are formed when a redundant fold of skin is compressed during the X-ray. In the case shown in **Figure 2.16**, the skin fold is adjacent to the scapula and can be confidently diagnosed if the line can be followed outside the thoracic cavity. Such lines often follow the breast folds, but these will also extend outside the chest.

Lesions on the skin (e.g. large warts, neurofibromas and benign breast masses) may also cause an apparent opacity on a PA chest X-ray. This occurs if the lesions are dense or

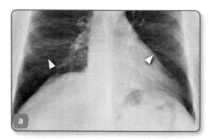

Figure 2.15 (a) Chest X-ray showing two small rounded nodules (arrowheads) in the lower zones. (b) The chest X-ray is repeated with wire clips (arrowheads) over the nipples, which confirms that the nodules correspond to the nipples.

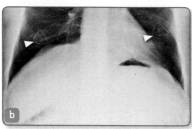

surrounded by air. If doubt exists about the cause, a lateral view, or a repeat with markers on the lesion (as is done with nipple markers), may confirm that the lesion is outside the lung.

Clinical insight

Lines from skin folds may be confused with the edge of a pneumothorax. However, awareness of their causes and appearance, as well as the presence of lung markings outside the line, should make the observer aware of the actual cause.

Mastectomy

Mastectomy can cause various apparent abnormalities. If the mastectomy is partial, the contour of the breast and axillary skin folds may be just mildly altered. If more complete, the reduction in soft tissue that the X-rays pass through makes the whole hemithorax appear more lucent (darker) (**Figure 2.17**).

A mastectomy may be replaced with an implant (**Figure 2.18**). Implants may be bilateral. They are usually denser than the original soft tissues, so may resemble a mass.

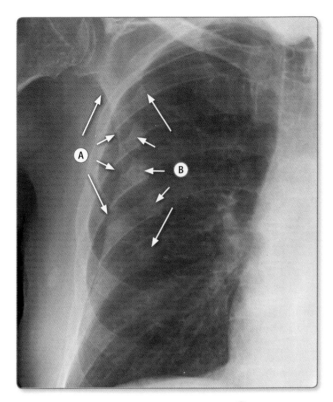

Figure 2.16 (a) Chest X-ray showing the line of a skin fold Ⓐ following the edge of the scapula. (b) An incidental finding is old healed rib fractures Ⓑ.

Body jewellery, hair and clothing

For a chest X-ray, patients should be dressed in a hospital gown and all extraneous objects that might cause an artefact on the film removed, if possible. Such items include objects in pockets, hair braids (**Figure 2.19**) that lie low over the body, and densities in clothing (e.g. sequins). Some objects, such as body jewellery (e.g. nipple rings, **Figure 2.20**) may not be removable

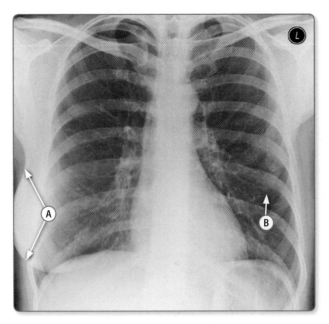

Figure 2.17 Chest X-ray showing left mastectomy. (A) Margins of right breast. (B) No skin edge of the left breast is visible. Also, the lower zone lung appears slightly darker than on the right because of decreased soft tissue for the X-ray beam to pass through.

but knowledge of their appearance should prevent mistakes in interpretation.

2.4 Systematic approach to reviewing the chest X-ray

Systematic review of any image in diagnostic radiology is essential to decide a final diagnosis. It is necessary to develop a routine for reviewing chest X-rays to avoid overlooking any information. Radiographers must know the appearance of a normal chest X-ray.

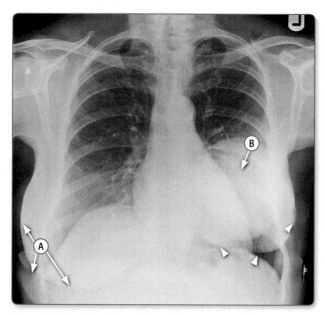

Figure 2.18 Chest X-ray showing left partial mastectomy with breast implant. (A) Contour of normal right breast. (B) Rounded opacity, the implant. Abnormal contour of left breast following surgery (arrowheads).

One effective systematic approach to reviewing the image is to consider each of the following characteristics in the order shown in **Table 2.1**.

Step 1: identification of the X-ray and clinical information

Before looking for any abnormality, it is essential to first check the patient's name, date of birth and date of examination and to confirm these on the X-ray. The clinical information provided is important in deciding a diagnosis. Mistaken patient identity can lead to serious mistakes.

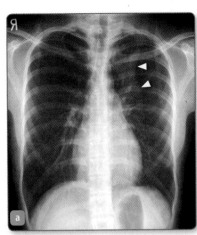

Figure 2.19 (a) Chest X-ray showing a soft tissue opacity (arrowheads) projected over the upper left chest. (b) The opacity disappears when the film is repeated with the patient's hair braid lifted out of the way.

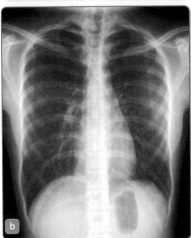

Step 2: checking technical factors

Positioning

Positioning should be ascertained, i.e. whether the X-ray is PA or anteroposterior (AP). The heart is magnified on the AP view,

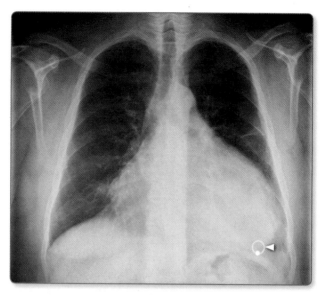

Figure 2.20 Chest X-ray showing a left nipple ring (arrowhead). Although obvious in this example, body jewellery can sometimes be mistaken for inhaled or ingested foreign bodies.

as described in Chapter 1. This can make assessment of possible cardiomegaly difficult (**Figure 2.21**).

Side markers

Identifying right or left is mandatory. Absent markers should be flagged to the radiographers before a report is issued.

Patient rotation

Patient rotation can distort the appearance of the mediastinum, or the lung lesions can be hidden behind the mediastinum. Rotation can also make one lung appear slightly denser than the other (**Figure 2.22**). The most common patient rotation is along a vertical axis. This can be assessed by looking at the

Step	Details
1. Identification	Identify: 1. the X-ray 2. the clinical information
2. Check technical factors	–
3. Examination	Examine the: 1. trachea and root of the neck 2. lung fields 3. silhouette sign 4. mediastinum and heart 5. fissures 6. hila 7. diaphragm and below the diaphragm 8. bones and so ft tissues 9. artefacts 10. abnormal densities
4. Diagnosis	–

Table 2.1 A systematic approach to reviewing a chest X-ray

distances of the medial ends of the clavicles from the vertebral spinous process at the same level. Without any rotation, these distances should be the same.

Degree of inspiration
Degree of inspiration can be gauged by counting the number of posterior ribs seen above the diaphragm. Ten are visible in a good inspiration. Alternatively, six should be visible if the anterior ends of the ribs are counted. Poor inspiratory effort can make the lower zones appear denser because these lung zones are underaerated. Heart size may also be difficult to judge on an underinspired X-ray (**Figure 2.23**).

Erect or supine position
The position of the patient can affect the appearance of an abnormality on X-ray. Erect X-rays are ideal, but very ill patients and babies are unable to have X-rays in the erect position. Awareness is essential because small pneumothoraces and

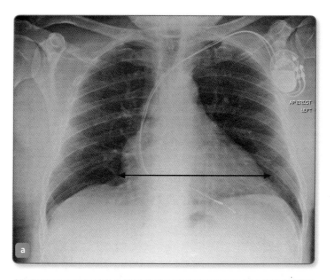

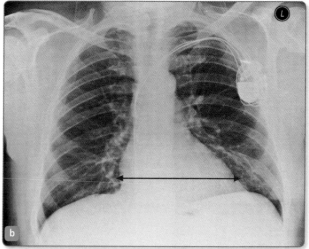

Figure 2.21 (a) AP chest X-ray showing marked cardiomegaly with increased transverse cardiac diameter (arrow). (b) PA view for the same patient. The heart appears smaller (diameter denoted by arrow); it was magnified in the AP view.

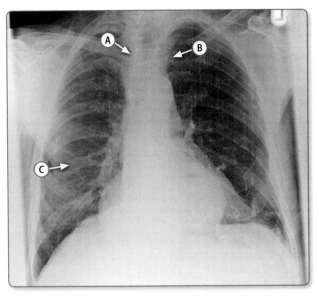

Figure 2.22 Chest X-ray showing patient rotation. The medial ends of the clavicles Ⓐ and Ⓑ are not equidistant from the spinous process. The right lung Ⓒ appears denser than the left because of the rotation.

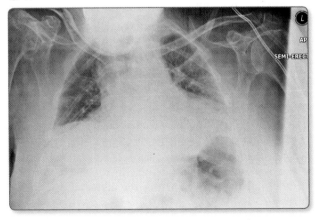

Figure 2.23 AP chest X-ray obtained in a semierect position with poor inspiratory effort. The lung bases aren't visible and there is apparent cardiomegaly.

air–fluid levels may be missed or misinterpreted on a supine X-ray.

Step 3: examination

Trachea and root of the neck

The trachea is usually central and filled with air, but it can be deviated slightly to the right around the aortic arch. Look for any narrowing, displacement or endotracheal lesions. The soft tissue on the right side of the trachea is known as the paratracheal stripe and is normally <5 mm thick. Adenopathy and other mediastinal mass lesions can increase paratracheal soft tissue. Assess the root of the neck for any large soft tissue causing tracheal deviation or narrowing, e.g. a large goitre.

Lung fields

Identify any increase or decrease in density and compare with the appearance of the opposite lung. Assess the lung markings or note their absence. On a PA X-ray, the diaphragm, heart and bones of the thoracic cage obscure a significant part of the lungs. Some of these hidden areas can be assessed by additional X-rays such as the lateral and AP views.

Silhouette sign

This term was coined by Felson to describe the loss of a normal radiographic border on a chest X-ray. The borders are usually lost by an adjacent opacity, and the silhouette sign is used to localise the site of the abnormality on an X-ray. This is dealt with in more detail in section 3.5.

Mediastinum and heart

The mediastinum is the opacity in the centre of the chest in a PA or an AP X-ray. The margins are normally sharp, except when prominent fat pads are adjacent to the inferior borders of the heart next to the diaphragm. The superior mediastinal contour in babies is widened by the normal thymus gland (**Figure 2.24**).

The heart occupies the mediastinum, with one third of it to the right of the midline and the other two thirds to the left.

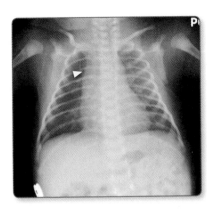

Figure 2.24 Chest X-ray showing normal thymus (arrowhead) in a neonate, causing widening of the superior mediastinum.

Measure the transverse cardiac diameter; the heart may appear larger in an AP X-ray (see **Figure 2.21**) or in poor inspiration (see **Figure 2.23**).

Fissures

Only the horizontal or minor fissure is seen in the right lung on a PA view. It appears as a fine, thin, opaque line from the lateral aspect of the 6th rib running medially to the hilum. The horizontal and oblique fissures are seen on a lateral view.

Hila

The hilar density is caused by the normal pulmonary arteries and veins. The normal hilar nodes and air-filled bronchi do not contribute to the normal hilar density.

The left hilum is higher than the right because the left pulmonary artery lies above the left main bronchus (**Figure 2.25**). Adenopathy or mass lesions in the hilar regions can increase the density or size of a hilum. Lobar atelectasis or fibrosis can displace the hilum towards the abnormality.

Diaphragm

On the chest X-ray, the hemidiaphragm on each side is dome-shaped, with the convexity directed upwards. The

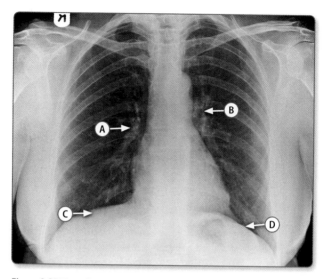

Figure 2.25 Normal posteroanterior chest X-ray showing the right hilum (A) lower than the left (B). The right hemidiaphragm (C) is higher than the left (D).

hemidiaphragms form acute angles laterally with the ribcage known as the costophrenic angles. The right hemidiaphragm is usually higher than the left (**Figure 2.25**).

The diaphragmatic outline is smooth and sharp, except where the heart sits on the diaphragm or where its outline is obliterated, i.e. in the centre of the diaphragm on an AP or a PA view, and the anterior aspect of the left hemidiaphragm on a lateral view. The outline of the diaphragm is obliterated pathologically on a chest X-ray in pleural effusions, lower lobe consolidation, atelectasis or any mass lesion in contact with the diaphragm.

Below the diaphragm

Check for any abnormality below the diaphragm. In a patient with normal situs, the liver appears as a soft tissue density under the right hemidiaphragm and cannot be separated from the diaphragmatic soft tissue. Air-filled stomach is often seen on the left.

Free intraperitoneal air appears as a curvilinear lucency under the diaphragm (**Figure 2.26**). Differentiate this condition from Chiladaiti syndrome, in which the bowel is interpositioned between the liver and diaphragm. Calcified gallstones and calcified granulomas under the diaphragm may be seen.

Bones and soft tissues

Systematically assess the bones and soft tissues of the thoracic cage, looking for any bony metastases or fractures (**Figure 2.27**).

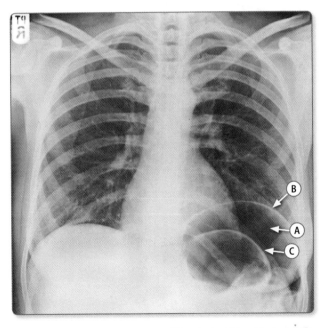

Figure 2.26 Chest X-ray showing free gas Ⓐ under the left hemidiaphragm Ⓑ in a patient with duodenal perforation. Ⓒ The air-filled fundus of the stomach.

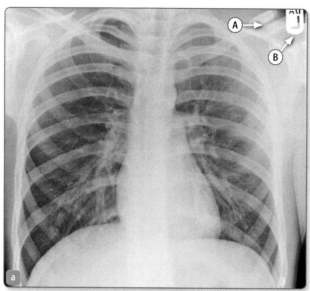

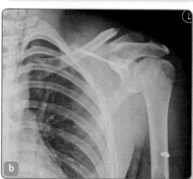

Figure 2.27 (a) Chest X-ray showing fracture (A) of the lateral shaft of the left clavicle visible at the edge of the X-ray. The fracture is almost obscured by the side marker (B) and can easily be missed. (b) Formal view of the shoulder of the same patient, showing fracture of the left clavicle.

Bony metastases may be visualised as sclerotic (dense) or lytic (lucent) lesions.

Soft tissues around the ribcage may show densities or calcification. Air is seen in the soft tissues in surgical or subcutaneous emphysema.

Artefacts

Artefacts from clothing, jewellery and skin folds can mimic pathological conditions. Awareness of various lines and tubes is essential. Artefacts are covered in section 2.3.

Abnormal densities

An abnormality may be an opacity or a lucency. Further characterisation and localisation is necessary, e.g. whether the abnormality is unilateral or bilateral and whether it affects a particular zone (see Chapter 3 for more).

Step 4: diagnosis

A diagnosis is made when all abnormalities have been assessed and considered in the context of the clinical information. Further views or imaging by other modalities may occasionally be necessary to come to a diagnosis. Systematic review of the chest X-ray ensures that all available data are scrutinised to help make the diagnosis.

Review areas

It is often essential to remember to examine areas that may be overlooked on first examination of the X-ray. These include the apices, the areas outside the thoracic cavity and below the diaphragm, and the shoulder joints (if included).

2.5 Postsurgical appearances

Pneumonectomy

Resection of a lung is most commonly done to treat lung cancer. In the 24 h after surgery, the empty hemithorax contains only air. It subsequently fills with fluid over the next few weeks, during which an air–fluid level is visible. By 4 months, the hemithorax should be completely opacified and the volume in the affected side reduced, resulting in ipsilateral mediastinal shift (**Figure 2.28**). Failure of mediastinal shift usually indicates complications, e.g. development of a bronchopleural fistula, empyema or haemorrhage.

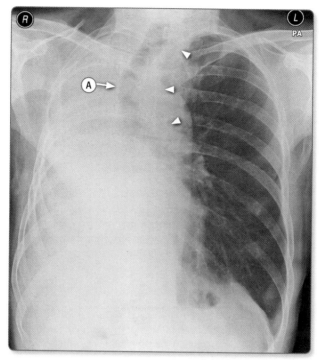

Figure 2.28 Chest X-ray showing right pneumonectomy 6 months after surgery. The trachea Ⓐ is deviated to the right, indicating significant volume loss, and is a reassuring sign. The right main bronchus is absent. The left lung is hyperinflated, resulting in hyperlucency and expansion of the left upper lobe across the midline into the right hemithorax Ⓑ.

Lobectomy

Lobar resection may be done for various malignant and non-malignant indications. The postsurgical appearances of lobectomy (e.g. left lower lobectomy, **Figure 2.29**) are similar to those of lobar atelectasis. This similarity results from the shift of mediastinal structures and development of a localised pleural effusion or fibrothorax opacifying the postlobectomy

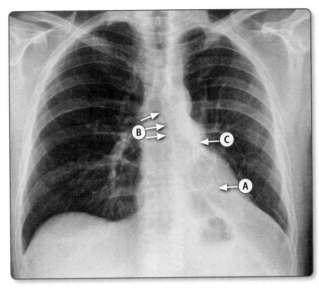

Figure 2.29 Chest X-ray showing left lower lobectomy. Volume loss is apparent in the left hemithorax, with slight crowding of the ribs, elevation of the left hemidiaphragm Ⓐ and displacement of the anterior mediastinal contents to the left Ⓑ. Depression of the hilar point Ⓒ indicates that the volume loss is in the left lower lobe. The left upper lobe has expanded to fill most of the hemithorax, resulting in sparsity of vessels.

bed, thus mimicking atelectatic lung. Identification of surgical clips or other evidence of surgical intervention may allow a confident distinction to be made.

Thoracotomy

Postsurgical evidence of thoracotomy in the absence of lung or lobe resection is often minimal, with absence of or damage to a rib the only sign of intervention (**Figure 2.30**).

Guiding principle

Using a systematic approach greatly lessens the chances of missing an abnormality.

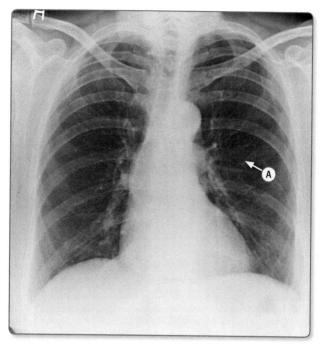

Figure 2.30 Chest X-ray showing left thoracotomy. Absence of the left 8th rib Ⓐ is the only indicator of previous surgery.

Coronary artery bypass graft

Coronary artery bypass grafting is done through a sternotomy. Metallic wires visible on the chest X-ray are used to close the chest wall. Surgical staples are used for fixing and positioning the grafts. These metallic structures are visible on the chest X-ray (**Figure 2.31**).

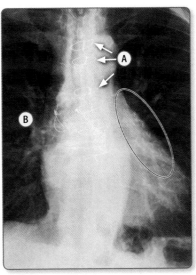

Figure 2.31 Chest X-ray showing sternotomy and coronary artery bypass graft clips. (A) Sternotomy wires in the midline. (B) A displaced wire. Multiple surgical staples are circled in the left anterior descending coronary artery territory.

Recognising abnormal signs

3.1 Lung opacities

Airspace opacification

Airspace opacification is otherwise known as alveolar opacification. It is caused by replacement of the alveolar air by fluid, cells or other material. The history will usually help differentiate between these entities. X-rays may show either a diffuse or a localised airspace disease. **Table 3.1** lists the causes of alveolar opacification.

Radiographic findings

The findings are unilateral or bilateral. The condition begins with small irregular, nodular or fluffy opacities, which then form more confluent opacification. Diffuse or patchy consolidation is often seen. Perihilar 'bat's wing' distribution (**Figure 3.1a**) is typical of pulmonary oedema but is also seen in other conditions (e.g. *Pneumocystis* pneumonia). The air bronchograms in **Figure 3.1a** and a computerised tomography (CT) scan (**Figure 3.1b**) are caused by air in the bronchi (black or grey) surrounded by consolidated lung. Airspace opacification can clear rapidly, within hours, in cardiac failure. In infection and haemorrhage, resolution is much slower.

Pulmonary masses

Various conditions can present as a pulmonary mass lesion on a chest X-ray (**Table 3.2**). The conditions may manifest as solitary or multiple pulmonary masses and can be benign or malignant.

Radiographic findings

A pulmonary mass (**Figure 3.2**) appears as an opacity >3 cm in diameter. Single or multiple masses may be visible. The masses may have irregular or smooth margins, depending on their nature. Abscesses may show areas of cavitation. Calcification

Cause	Example(s)
Exudate	Infection (bacterial, viral or fungal)
	Aspiration
Transudate	Cardiac failure
	Acute respiratory distress syndrome
	Hypoproteinaemia
	Any cause of fluid overload
Blood	Trauma
	Vasculitis
	Haemosiderosis
Cells	Alveolar cell carcinoma
	Metastases
	Lymphoproliferative infiltration
Other	Alveolar proteinosis

Table 3.1 Causes of alveolar opacification

is often seen in granulomas and hamartomas but these are usually smaller.

Pulmonary nodules

Macronodular opacities

Nodules are rounded opacities of <3 cm. Macronodular opacities are usually defined as nodules >5 mm in diameter. Nodules may contain cavitation or calcification. Multiple nodules are seen in various conditions (**Table 3.3**).

Radiographic findings The nodular lesions are often rounded with smooth or irregular margins. The density, distribution, size and other associated radiological findings allow diagnosis.
- Cavitation is seen in abscesses or cavitating metastases.
- Metastases usually have smooth margins but vary in size (**Figure 3.3**).

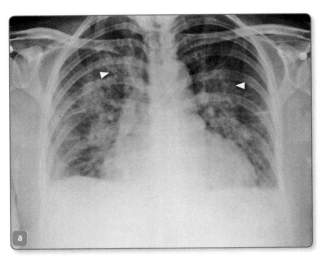

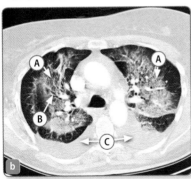

Figure 3.1 (a) Chest X-ray showing opacification of the bilateral perihilar air space in a bat's wing distribution (arrowheads) typical of pulmonary oedema. (b) Computerised tomography scan of the same patient, showing pulmonary oedema with perihilar air space opacification (A), air bronchograms (B) and bilateral pleural effusions (C).

- Sarcoid and pneumoconioses have nodules of about the same size.
- Sarcoid nodules tend to be perihilar and in the upper zones.
- Rheumatoid nodules are most often in the lower zones.
- Calcified hilar nodes are seen with sarcoid, silicosis and tuberculosis.

Cause	Examples
Malignant lesions	Squamous cell, small cell or adenocarcinoma lung cancer
	Sarcoma
	Pulmonary lymphoma
	Melanoma
	Metastatic lung lesions
Benign conditions	
Infections and infestations	Pneumonia
	Lung abscesses
	Hydatid cysts
	Aspergilloma (fungal ball)
	Granulomas
Congenital	Arteriovenous malformation
	Bronchogenic cyst
	Sequestration
Other	Pulmonary infarct
	Lung contusion or haematoma
	Round atelectasis
	Pulmonary artery aneurysm
	Bronchial carcinoid
	Focal scarring or massive fibrosis in pneumoconioses

Table 3.2 Differential diagnosis of pulmonary masses

Small nodular opacities

Small nodular opacities are nodules of 2–5 mm. They may be single or multiple. Some of the causes of small nodules are the same as those of micro- and macronodular disease.

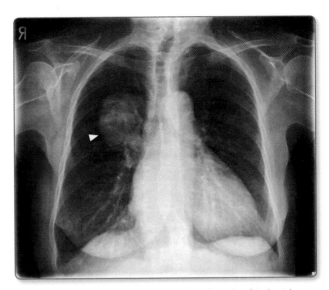

Figure 3.2 Chest X-ray showing a pulmonary mass (arrowhead) in the right upper zone, later diagnosed as a bronchogenic carcinoma.

Cause	Examples
Metastases	Metastases arising in breast, lung, kidney or gastrointestinal tract
Infection	Tuberculosis
	Abscesses
	Fungal infection
Collagen vascular disease	Rheumatoid arthritis
	Wegener granulomatosis
Pneumoconiosis	Silicosis
Other	Sarcoid, amyloid and arteriovenous malformations

Table 3.3 Differential diagnosis of macronodular opacities

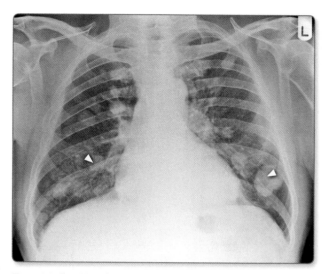

Figure 3.3 Chest X-ray showing multiple nodules of varying sizes (arrowheads) in both lungs. These are metastases from renal cell carcinoma, often referred to as cannon ball metastases.

Tuberculosis, sarcoid, and metastases from thyroid, breast and melanoma all give rise to small nodules. Other causes of multiple small nodular opacities are eosinophilic granulomas, hypersensitivity pneumonitis, histiocytosis and pulmonary oedema. Previous chickenpox (varicella pneumonia, **Figure 3.4**), histoplasmosis, coccidioidomycosis and old tuberculosis give rise to multiple small calcified nodules.

Radiographic findings
Chest X-rays and CT scans show small, rounded and occasionally calcified opacities. Nodules of metastases, tuberculosis, granulomas and sarcoid are more discrete than the poorly defined or confluent opacities seen in pulmonary oedema.

Micronodular opacities
Micronodular opacities are often interchangeably referred to as miliary nodules. Micronodules are 0.5–1 mm, whereas miliary

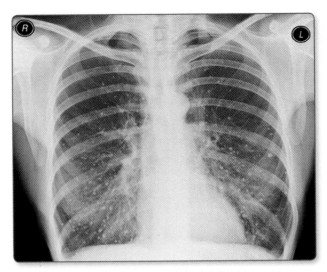

Figure 3.4 Chest X-ray showing multiple small calcified nodular opacities secondary to old varicella pneumonia.

nodules may be up to 2 mm in diameter. However, in practice micronodules are essentially those measuring 0.5–2 mm. **Table 3.4** lists their main causes.

Radiographic findings The nodules appear as fine pin-point opacities or miliary opacities. These opacities are widespread in the lungs in miliary tuberculosis (**Figure 3.5 and 3.6**) and histoplasmosis, and they have no zonal predominance.

Sarcoid usually has a perihilar distribution. Rarely, it has a widespread miliary appearance. High-density fine nodules are seen in silicosis and other heavy metal inhalational diseases (e.g. stannosis and berylliosis). In silicosis, nodules tend to be distributed in the upper zones and may have calcified mediastinal and hilar nodes, usually in an eggshell pattern of calcification of the nodes. Associated upper zone fibrosis is often present.

Type	Causes
Widespread, soft tissue density	Miliary tuberculosis (**Figure 3.5**) and histoplasmosis, both caused by disseminated haematogenous spread and difficult to differentiate
	Sarcoid, hypersensitivity pneumonitis and panbronchiolitis (**Figure 3.6**)
Miliary metastases	Thyroid carcinoma and melanoma
High-density micronodules	Silicosis, haemosiderosis, berylliosis and stannosis

Table 3.4 Types and causes of micronodular opacities

Cavitating lesions

A cavitation in the lung is an area of transradiancy surrounded by opacification or wall. Cavitating lesions may be either a ring lesion or a cavity or transradiancy in an area of consolidation or mass. Assessment of the size, site, number, wall thickness, margins and intracavitary contents of the lesions helps differentiate the cause (**Table 3.5**).

> **Clinical insight**
>
> *Miliary* means 'resembling millet seeds'. Miliary nodules should be evenly distributed, without a zonal predominance.

Radiographic findings A cavitating lesion is generally seen as a ring lesion with central lucency, with or without an air–fluid level.

- Cavitating lesions are thick-walled and irregular in carcinoma (**Figure 3.7**) and tuberculosis.
- They are multiple in metastases, Wegener granulomatosis and rheumatoid arthritis (**Figure 3.8**).
- They are multiple with thin walls in staphylococcal pneumatocoeles.
- An intracavitatory mass may indicate an aspergilloma, tumour or clot and often has as an air crescent sign, particularly in aspergillomas.

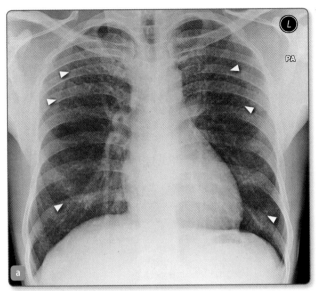

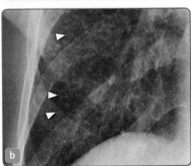

Figure 3.5 (a) Chest X-ray showing widespread fine miliary nodules (arrowheads) in both lungs in a patient with miliary tuberculosis. (b) Magnified image of (a) showing multiple micronodules (arrowheads) in tuberculosis.

3.2 Atelectasis

Atelectasis is partial or complete loss of volume, i.e. collapse, of the lung. Partial atelectasis may be lobar (involving the whole lobe), segmental or subsegmental. **Table 3.6** lists the causes of atelectasis.

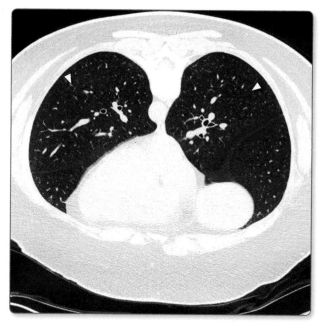

Figure 3.6 Prone computerised tomography scan showing multiple fine branching micronodular opacities (arrowheads) in a patient with extensive bronchiolitis.

Types of atelectasis

There are four types of atelectasis.

- Obstructive or resorption atelectasis: secondary to a foreign body, mucus or tumour (**Figure 3.9**).
- Passive atelectasis: a large pleural effusion or mass, pneumothorax, diaphragmatic paralysis or rupture.
- Cicatrisation atelectasis (caused by scarring): seen after infections, particularly tuberculosis, and in sarcoid and pulmonary fibrosis.
- Adhesive atelectasis: caused by loss of alveolar surfactant (i.e. respiratory distress syndrome).

Cause	Example(s)
Infections	Klebsiella
	Staphylococcus
	Tuberculosis
	Fungal infection
Tumours	Squamous cell lung cancer
	Metastases
Vascular	Pulmonary infarcts
	Septic emboli
	Wegener granulomatosis (vasculitis)
Connective tissue disorders	Rheumatoid arthritis
Trauma	Laceration of lung
	Cysts

Table 3.5 Differential diagnosis of cavitating lesions

Radiographic findings

Atelectasis shows general signs of lack of aeration of the involved lung and displacement of fissures, hilum and diaphragm. The sections below cover more specific signs for individual lobar and segmental atelectasis on X-ray.

Whole lung atelectasis

Any of the above-mentioned causes of atelectasis can cause atelectasis of the whole lung.

Radiographic findings

The chest X-ray shows complete opacification (white-out) and loss of volume of the affected hemithorax. The loss of volume is evidenced by deviation of the trachea and mediastinum to the side of the atelectasis and crowding of the ribs on the affected side (**Figure 3.9**).

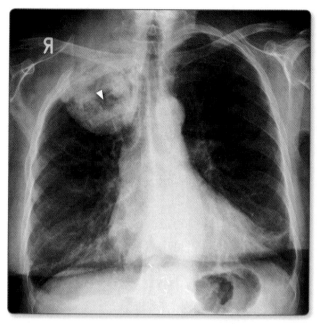

Figure 3.7 Chest X-ray showing large Pancoast tumour (arrowhead)in the right upper zone with central cavitation. The first two ribs on the right have been destroyed by the tumour.

Lobar atelectasis
Radiographic findings

Right upper lobe atelectasis The horizontal fissure rises upwards, depending on the degree of right upper lobe atelectasis, and becomes more vertical. This effect is best seen on posteroanterior (PA) X-rays (**Figure 3.10**). The fissure may even be concave inferiorly. The atelectatic lobe lacks air and becomes more opaque. The oblique fissure is more vertical and is visualised on lateral view as the posterior margin of the wedge-shaped opacity (**Figure 3.11**). The trachea is often deviated to the right. The right hilum and right hemidiaphragm

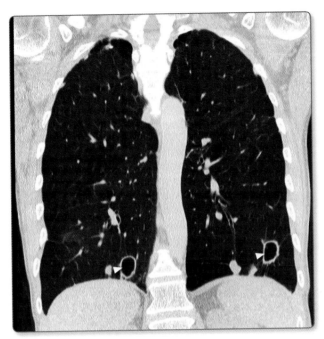

Figure 3.8 Reformatted coronal computerised tomography scan showing cavitating lower zone nodules (arrowheads) in rheumatoid disease.

are elevated. There may be compensatory hyperinflation of the middle and lower lobes, which may be more lucent. CT is useful to assess the cause of the atelectasis.

Right middle lobe atelectasis This is better visualised on a lateral view, on which it appears a narrow triangular opacity with its apex in the hilum (**Figure 3.12**). The oblique and horizontal fissures move closer to each other. On the PA view, this may be an ill-defined opacification adjacent to the heart, and the right heart border is almost always obscured by the right middle lobe atelectasis (**Figure 3.13**). The upper margin of the atelectasis sometimes appears as a straight line, i.e. the

Type of atelectasis	Causes	Examples
Endoluminal obstruction	Tumour	Bronchogenic carcinoma
		Metastases from breast, melanoma, colon and kidney
		Carcinoid
	Mucus	–
	Foreign body	–
	Infection or inflammation	Tuberculous granulomas
		Sarcoid granulomas
		Wegener granulomatosis
	Other	Amyloid
		Broncholith
Extrinsic compression of airways or lung	Adenopathy	Lymphoma
		Metastases
		Tuberculosis
		Sarcoid
	Other	Large pleural effusion
		Scarring
		Cardiomegaly
		Pleural tumours
		Pneumothorax

Table 3.6 Causes of atelectasis

horizontal fissure. The right middle lobe atelectasis may be unclear on the PA X-ray.

Lower lobe atelectasis Both lower lobes lose volume in a similar fashion. The atelectatic lower lobe moves posteriorly, medially and inferiorly.

On the PA view, the atelectasis is a triangular density with its base on the medial aspect of the hemidiaphragm. On the left, the atelectasis overlies the cardiac shadow (**Figure 3.14**);

on the right, it appears to the right of the midline. The lower lobe atelectasis does not obliterate the cardiac margins, which are projected through the atelectatic lobe, and causes downward displacement of the ipsilateral hilum.

On the lateral X-ray, the lower lobe atelectasis is a triangular density posteriorly and inferiorly. The oblique fissure is displaced downwards and to the back (**Figure 3.15**).

Left upper lobe atelectasis Atelectasis of the left upper lobe appears as an ill-defined veil-like opacification radiating from the left hilum and obliterating the cardiac margin on the left (**Figure 3.16**). This differs from the appearance of atelectasis

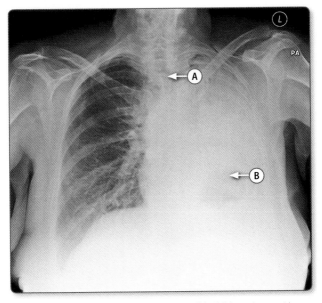

Figure 3.9 Chest X-ray showing total white-out of the left hemithorax, with loss of volume caused by atelectasis of the left lung and with mediastinal and tracheal (A) shift to the left. Elevation of the left hemidiaphragm is visible as raised gastric air bubbles (B). The left ribs are crowded.

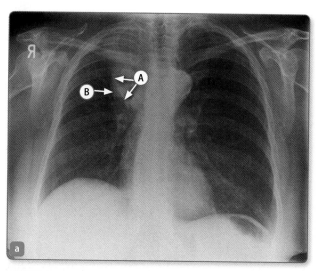

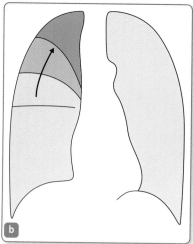

Figure 3.10 (a) Chest X-ray showing right upper lobe atelectasis caused by a tumour. The atelectatic upper lobe appears as a wedge-shaped opacity in the right apex. The straight lateral border of this opacity is the elevated horizontal fissure (A). The overlying bulging and rounded opacity (B) at the inferior aspect is tumour. (b) Right upper lobe atelectasis (arrow) on a posteroanterior view.

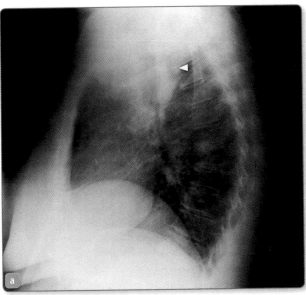

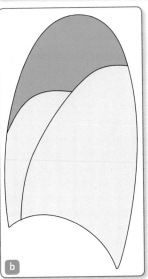

Figure 3.11 (a) Lateral X-ray of right upper lobe atelectasis, showing elevation of an oblique fissure (arrowhead), seen as a straight margin posterior to the wedge opacity of the atelectatic right upper lobe in the apex. (b) Lateral view of right upper lobe atelectasis.

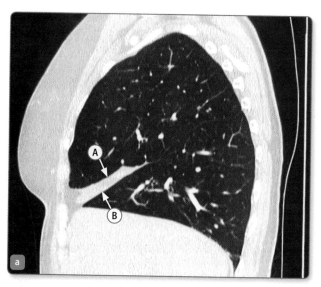

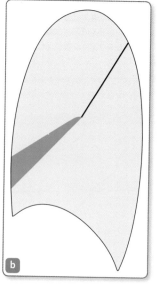

Figure 3.12 (a) Reformatted sagittal–lateral computerised tomography scan showing right middle lobe atelectasis. The straight upper margin of the wedge opacity is the horizontal fissure Ⓐ and the lower margin the oblique fissure Ⓑ. (b) Right middle lobe atelectasis in lateral view.

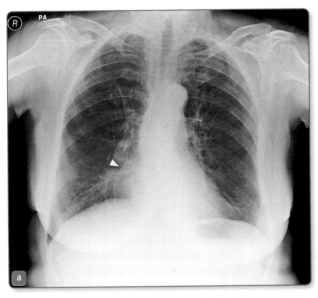

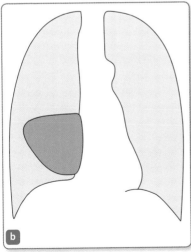

Figure 3.13 (a) PA X-ray showing right middle lobe atelectasis as irregular opacification adjacent to and obscuring the right heart border (arrowhead). (b) Right middle lobe atelectasis in a PA view.

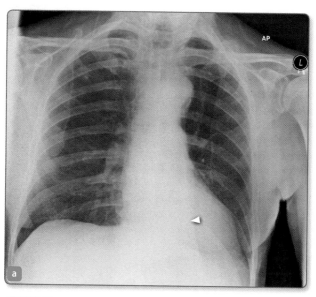

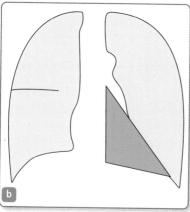

Figure 3.14 (a) Chest X-ray showing left lower lobe atelectasis as a triangular density (arrowhead) overlying the cardiac shadow. The medial aspect of the left hemidiaphragm is obliterated by the atelectasis. (b) Left lower lobe atelectasis on a posteroanterior view.

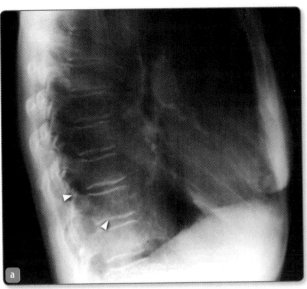

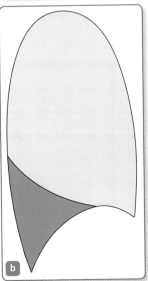

Figure 3.15 (a) Lateral X-ray view of left lower lobe atelectasis. The oblique fissure has been displaced downwards and to the back (arrowheads). The lower thoracic vertebrae show increased opacification caused by overlying lower lobe atelectasis. The lower thoracic vertebrae are normally more lucent (black) because of the aerated lungs. (b) Left lower lobe atelectasis on a lateral view.

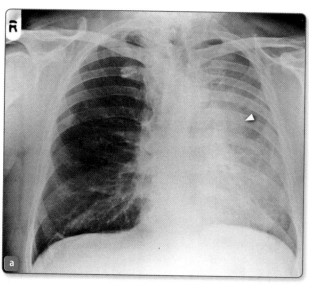

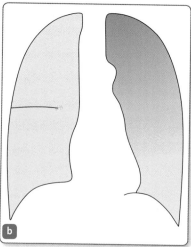

Figure 3.16 (a) Chest X-ray showing left upper lobe atelectasis as a veil-like opacification of the left hemithorax (arrowhead), obliterating the left cardiac margin but not the hemidiaphragm. Lucency around the aortic knuckle is caused by compensatory hyperinflation of the lower lobe. (b) Left upper lobe atelectasis in the posteroanterior view.

of the right upper lobe because of the presence of lingula on the left. The upper mediastinum is shifted to the left and the left hilum often elevated. The atelectatic left upper lobe moves anteriorly and is just behind the sternum. On the lateral view (**Figure 3.17**), the oblique fissure runs parallel to the sternum. Compensatory hyperinflation of the left lower lobe appears as a band of lucency running parallel to the sternum between the atelectatic left upper lobe and sternum. The hyperinflation may also manifest as lucency around the aortic knuckle, i.e. the Luftsichel sign, on the PA view (**Figure 3.16**). The left hemidiaphragm is not obscured by left upper lobe atelectasis.

Linear atelectasis

Linear atelectasis, also known as plate or discoid atelectasis, is focal loss of lung volume mainly at a subsegmental level. As the name implies, it appears as a linear opacity commonly in the lung bases, parallel to the diaphragm. These lines are several centimetres long and 1–3 mm thick. Most extend to the pleura and run horizontally but some are seen in the oblique or vertical plane.

Mechanism

Linear atelectasis is a non-obstructive atelectasis that can be caused by underaeration of a subsegment of the lung, most often in the lung bases secondary to impaired diaphragmatic excursion. Underaeration is seen in patients who have had surgery or general anaesthesia or who have painful abdominal conditions or masses. A less common cause is lack of surfactant causing reduced compliance secondary to ischaemia, e.g. in pulmonary embolism.

Radiographic findings

On chest X-ray and CT scan, linear atelectasis appears as a linear or thin band of opacification extending from the pleura. The opacification is usually in the lung bases, parallel to the diaphragm (**Figure 3.18**).

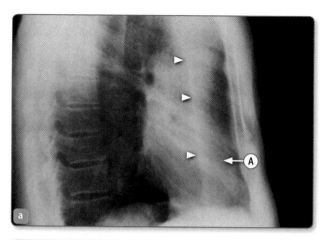

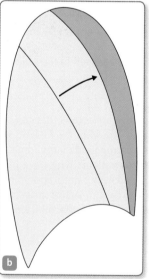

Figure 3.17 (a) Lateral X-ray view of left upper lobe atelectasis. The oblique fissure is parallel to and just behind the sternum, seen as a vertical line (arrowheads). Anterior to the oblique fissure is the atelectatic left upper lobe, seen as a band of opacification (arrowhead). Behind the fissure is the hyperinflated left lower lobe. (b) Lateral view of left upper lobe atelectasis.

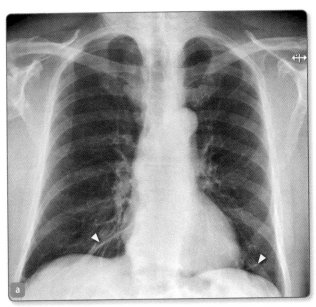

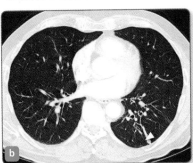

Figure 3.18 Linear atelectasis. (a) Chest X-ray showing linear opacities (arrowheads) in the lung bases extending from the pleura. (b) Axial computerised tomography scan showing a thin linear opacity (arrowhead) in the left lower lobe extending to the pleura.

Round atelectasis

Round atelectasis (folded lung or Blesovsky syndrome) is a focal, pleural-based and uncommon type of lung atelectasis. It appears as a subpleural mass with ill-defined margins

(**Figure 3.19**). Round atelectasis is usually secondary to chronic pleural irritation and scarring. Most cases are seen in asbestos-related pleural disease. Tuberculous empyema causing pleural scarring can also lead to round atelectasis. Anatomically, round atelectasis is a non-segmental atelectasis.

Mechanism
Round atelectasis develops secondary to pleural effusion with associated chronic pleural inflammation. The exact mechanism of the development of round atelectasis is uncertain. It is most commonly believed to be caused by an area of focal subpleural atelectasis trapped in the visceral pleura by fibrinous adhesions or chronic pleural disease.

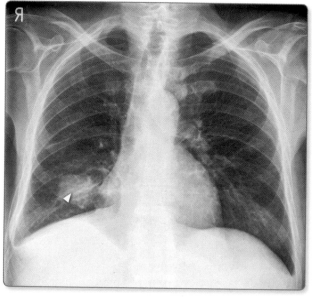

Figure 3.19 Chest X-ray showing a round mass (arrowhead) in the right lower zone, suggesting a tumour.

Radiographic findings

Round atelectasis appears on a CT scan (**Figure 3.20**) as a rounded subpleural mass with a comet tail appearance of

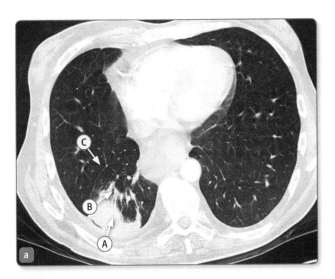

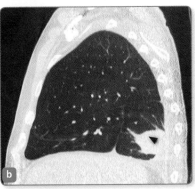

Figure 3.20 CT scans of same patient as Figure 3.19. (a) Axial scan confirms round atelectasis and volume loss in right lower lobe (A). Vessels and bronchi entering the subpleural mass (B) have a comet tail appearance. Oblique fissure is displaced medially (C). (b) Sagittal reformatted scan of round atelectasis in right lower lobe (arrowhead).

vessels and bronchi swirling into it in a spiral fashion. Signs of loss of volume are present. Other evidence of asbestos exposure is often seen as pleural plaques or thickening. Round atelectasis is usually at the lung bases posteromedially. An air bronchogram may occasionally be present in the mass. The mass can be difficult to distinguish from a tumour on a chest X-ray (**Figure 3.19**).

Management
Round atelectasis can mimic tumours on a chest X-ray, so further imaging by CT is essential. CT confirms the diagnosis in most cases. Further follow-up CT scans may occasionally be needed. If the imaging features on CT are consistent with round atelectasis, then it is managed conservatively.

3.3 Reticular opacities

Reticular opacities are lace-like opacities or interlacing linear opacities often referred to as reticulations (**Figure 3.21**). The opacities result from thickening of the interstitium of the lung (**Table 3.7**), i.e. the interlobular interstitial septa. Fine or coarse reticulations occur in various acute and chronic conditions.

Radiographic findings
The reticular opacities are best visualised on CT as a network of fine or coarse linear opacities that are interlaced (**Figure 3.22**).
- Smooth interstitial thickening is seen in cardiac failure, interstitial pneumonia and connective tissue disorders.
- Some reticular opacities are rapidly reversible (e.g. after treatment for cardiac failure) and some may resolve more slowly (e.g. in cases of infection, hypersensitivity pneumonitis and some idiopathic pneumonias).
- Several conditions produce persistent reticular opacities, some of which progress to honeycombing.
- Fine nodular or coarse reticulations are seen in lymphangitis (**Figure 3.21**), sarcoid and usual interstitial pneumonia on X-rays or CT scans.

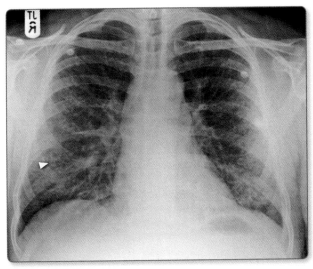

Figure 3.21 Chest X-ray showing reticular opacities in both lungs, best seen in the bases (arrowhead). Some reticulonodular opacities are also visible in this patient with lymphangitis.

Pathological change	Causes
Increased pulmonary venous pressure	Cardiac failure
	Venous obstructive disease
Lymphatic obstruction	Lymphangitis carcinomatosa
	Sarcoid
	Congenital lymphangiectasia
Accumulation of inflammatory or tumour cells in interstitium	Infections
	Interstitial pneumonias
	Connective tissue disorders
	Fibrosis
	Hypersensitivity pneumonitis
	Tumour infiltration
	Sarcoid
	Amyloidosis

Table 3.7 Mechanisms and causes of interstitial thickening and reticular opacities

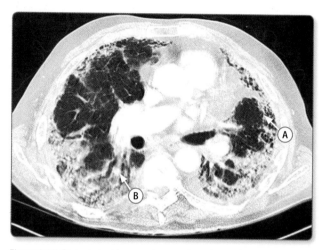

Figure 3.22 Computerised tomography scan of a patient with interstitial fibrosis, showing lace-like reticular opacities Ⓐ and traction bronchial dilatation Ⓑ secondary to the fibrosis and loss of volume.

- The reticular opacities on chest X-rays occur particularly in the lung bases and may make the cardiac outline appear shaggy.
- Zonal predominance occurs: lower zone involvement in idiopathic pulmonary fibrosis, rheumatoid lung and asbestosis, and upper zone predominance in sarcoidosis and ankylosing spondylitis.
- Loss of volume is another feature of fibrosis on both chest X-rays and CT scans.

Honeycombing

Honeycombing is end-stage interstitial fibrosis. It appears as coarse reticular opacities with cysts, loss of normal interstitial architecture and loss of volume (**Figure 3.23**). Honeycombing is present in idiopathic pulmonary fibrosis, connective tissue disorders, sarcoid, hypersensitivity pneumonitis, pneumoconiosis (asbestosis and silicosis), chronic aspiration and radiotherapy.

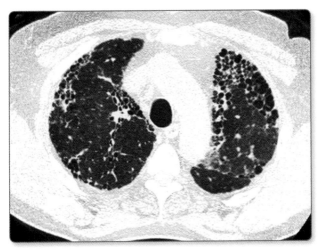

Figure 3.23 Computerised tomography scan showing honeycombing (arrowhead) as cystic areas with loss of normal architecture in a patient with fibrosis.

3.4 Pleural abnormalities

Pleural plaques

The presence of pleural plaques on a chest X-ray means that the patient has been exposed to asbestos. Pleural plaques take about 12 years to develop and be identified on a chest X-ray, and it usually takes 20 years or more for them to calcify. The extent of pleural plaques is dose-related and underestimated by radiological imaging. The sensitivity of a chest X-ray in detecting their presence is low (30–80%), but detection rates increase with the number and size of the plaques present.

> **Clinical insight**
>
> Looking at old chest X-rays is often useful because plaques grow slowly and will often be present on previous films.

Radiographic findings

Pleural plaques tend to spare the upper zones and costophrenic angles. The plaques almost always involve the parietal pleura but occasionally appear in the interlobular fissures. Calcified plaques viewed en face have stippled calcifications of uneven density (**Figures 3.24 and 3.25**).

Management

Pleural plaques do not tend to cause disability or pain and do not undergo malignant change. However, they inform the physician that the patient has been exposed to asbestos and is at increased risk of developing cancers such as mesothelioma.

> ### Clinical insight
>
> Always confirm the presence of pleural fluid with ultrasound before any pleural procedure (**Figure 3.26**).

> ### Clinical insight
>
> To differentiate between a raised hemidiaphragm and an effusion, look at the shape of the upper border. If the peak is lateral, it is likely to be pleural fluid.

Pleural effusions

Chest X-rays are useful when investigating possible pleural disease. Obtain a PA chest X-ray whenever possible.

In the healthy lung, normal pleura is visualised only where the visceral pleura invaginates into the lung to form a fissure. Pleural effusions are detected on clinical examination by reduced or absent breath sounds and a stony, dull percussion note.

Radiographic findings: Pleural fluid tends to collect along dependent surfaces, and blunting of the costophrenic angle is often the first sign of the accumulation of pleural fluid. At least 250 mL of pleural fluid needs to be present to be visible.

A meniscus sign is often seen on a standard PA chest X-ray, with homogeneous lower zone opacity and a concave upward sloping seen laterally. A large effusion can cause mediastinal shift, pushing the major airways away from the side of the effusion (**Figure 3.27**).

Subpulmonary effusion

Fluid may collect in a subpulmonary location. Subpulmonary effusion more commonly occurs on the right. The hemidiaphragm

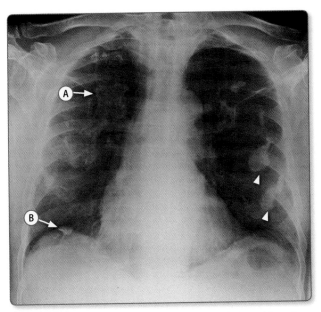

Figure 3.24 Chest X-ray showing multiple calcified pleural plaques bilaterally. (A) 'Holly leaf' calcification, (B) calcified diaphragmatic pleural plaque, arrowheads show calcified pleural plaques.

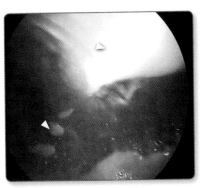

Figure 3.25
Thoracoscopic image showing calcified pleural plaques (arrowheads).

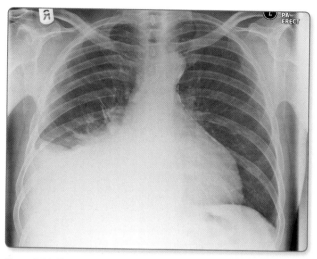

Figure 3.26 Chest X-ray showing moderate right pleural effusion secondary to heart failure. The cardiac shadow is enlarged.

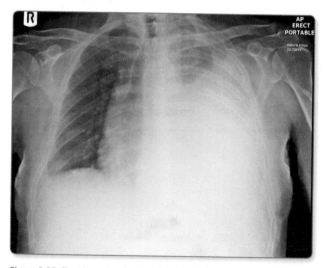

Figure 3.27 Chest X-ray showing large left pleural effusion with mediastinal shift.

is elevated; its medial aspect is flattened and the peak of the diaphragm displaced laterally. The costophrenic angle is usually ill defined.

Supine pleural effusion

Pleural fluid will layer posteriorly and can be easily missed in the supine position, appearing as an increased haziness over the lower zones (**Figure 3.28**). An apical cap can occur if the effusion is moderate to large.

Loculated pleural effusion

Loculated effusions do not move freely within the pleural space and occur when adhesions have formed between the visceral and parietal pleura (**Figure 3.29**). These effusions are commonly seen in cases of pleural infection.

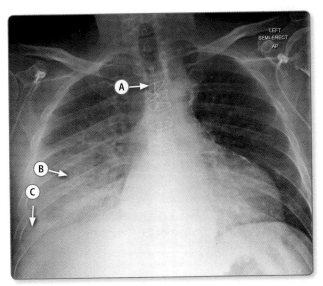

Figure 3.28 Supine plain chest X-ray showing pleural effusion. Poststernotomy wires Ⓐ and pleural fluid Ⓑ tracking posteriorly and causing hazy opacification Ⓒ. The pleural fluid causes loss of the costophrenic angle.

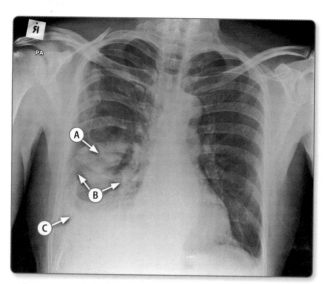

Figure 3.29 Chest X-ray showing loculated right-sided pleural effusion Ⓐ caused by an empyema. Ⓑ Chest tube in pleural cavity. Ⓒ Loss of the costophrenic angle caused by presence of pleural fluid.

Loculated effusions often have a sharp medial margin and a hazy lateral margin, with the margins making an obtuse angle with the chest wall. Thoracic ultrasound allows identification of septations and loculations, as well as a suitable site for chest drain insertion or fluid sampling.

Pleural thickening

Distinguishing pleural thickening from a small basal effusion is often difficult on a chest X-ray. It is often easier to identify pleural thickening on the lateral chest walls. If present, pleural thickening appears as a thickened white line around the lung edge.

If there is a smooth contour, bilateral and associated with pleural plaques, the diagnosis is highly likely to be diffuse pleural thickening secondary to asbestos exposure. Unilateral pleural thickening that appears nodular suggests underlying pleural malignancy. Malignant pleural thickening will often also cause loss of lung volume (**Figure 3.30**).

If the thickening is calcified, it often becomes more evident. Causes of calcified pleural thickening include asbestos exposure, previous pleural tuberculosis, previous empyema and long-standing residual haemothorax.

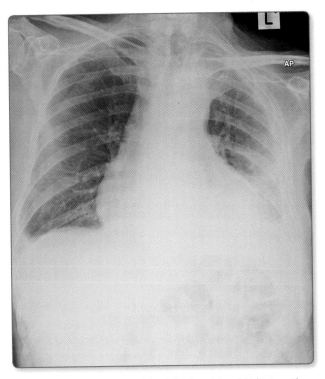

Figure 3.30 Chest X-ray showing left-sided unilateral pleural thickening with loss of volume in a patient with mesothelioma. The cardiac shadow is enlarged. CT confirmed pericardial effusion secondary to the malignancy.

Pneumothorax

Pneumothorax literally means 'air in the chest cavity'. It can be primary (occurring in a person with normal underlying lung) or secondary (associated with underlying lung disease, e.g. chronic obstructive pulmonary disease, interstitial lung disease and cystic fibrosis). Common symptoms include sudden onset of breathlessness, often associated with pleuritic chest discomfort.

Pneumothorax is also classified by measurement on PA plain chest X-ray. The 2010 British Thoracic Society guidelines recommend measuring the interpleural distance at the level of the hilum, between the edge of lung and the lateral chest wall (**Figure 3.31**). A measurement of >2 cm is classified as a large pneumothorax. The American College of Chest Physicians (ACCP) guidelines recommend measuring the distance between apex and cupola (**Figure 3.31**).

Clinical insight
Small apical pneumothorax can easily be missed. Take special care when trying to exclude this diagnosis, especially when viewing a chest X-ray on a suboptimal computer screen in a brightly lit medical ward.

Radiographic findings

A chest X-ray is always needed to confirm the diagnosis. Although inspiratory and expiratory films used to be advised, this is no longer felt to be beneficial.

On a normal chest X-ray, vascular lung markings are usually seen spreading to the periphery of the lung fields. No vascular markings are visible beyond the lung edge in a pneumothorax (**Figure 3.32**).

3.5 Mediastinal abnormalities

The chest X-ray provides a two-dimensional image of a three-dimensional structure. Mediastinal masses are recognised by the presence of distortion of the mediastinal contours. This is one factor that allows them to be distinguished from lung masses (see below). The clinician must rely on anatomical landmarks to

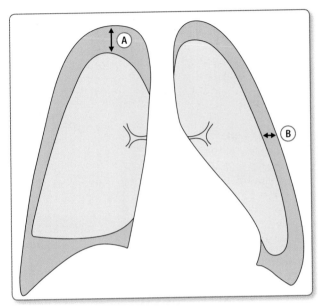

Figure 3.31 How to determine the size of a pneumothorax. Ⓐ Apex-to-cupola distance (American guidelines). Ⓑ Interpleural distance at the level of the hilum (British guidelines).

accurately localise a lesion and then narrow the list of differential diagnoses.

Analysis of mediastinal masses

Analysis of mediastinal masses involves a number of steps.

1. Distinguish mediastinal from pulmonary pathological conditions.
2. Locate the lesion in the mediastinum using the silhouette and other signs (see below).
3. Formulate a differential diagnosis based on the position of the mass.
4. Further imaging is usually needed to clarify the nature of the mass.

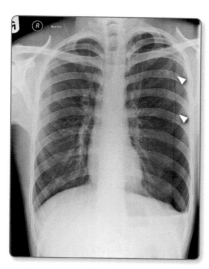

Figure 3.32 Chest X-ray showing left-sided spontaneous pneumothorax in a young man. The visceral pleura is visible (arrowheads). More laterally, lung markings are missing. Arrowheads point to the visceral pleura and edge of the atelectatic lung.

Guiding principle

Dr Benjamin Felson coined the term *silhouette sign* after reasoning that, 'An intrathoracic lesion touching a border of the heart, aorta, or diaphragm will obliterate that border. An intrathoracic lesion not anatomically contiguous with a border of one of these structures will not obliterate that border.'

Distinguishing mediastinal from lung masses

Mediastinal masses do not contain air bronchograms. They may distort the ribs, sternum or spine and form oblique angles with the lung rather than acute angles (**Figures 3.33 and 3.34**).

Mediastinal divisions

The mediastinum is arbitrarily divided into three compartments (**Figure 3.35**) to help develop differential diagnoses. Pathological conditions arise in structures in these compartments.

- The anterior mediastinum contains the thymus, lymph nodes, vessels and fat.
- The middle mediastinum contains the trachea, arch of aorta, great vessels, pulmonary arteries, oesophagus and lymph nodes.

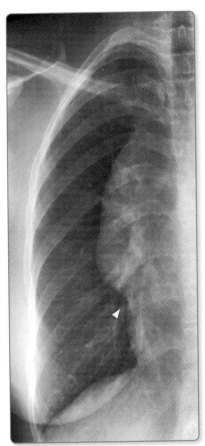

Figure 3.33 Chest X-ray showing large mediastinal mass (anterior) creating oblique angles (arrowhead) with the mediastinal contour.

- The posterior mediastinum contains nerve roots, the descending aorta and the vertebral column.

The silhouette sign

The silhouette sign is the loss of a normal radiographic border between two structures. It is a fundamental tool for anatomically localising pathological changes on a chest X-ray. The silhouette

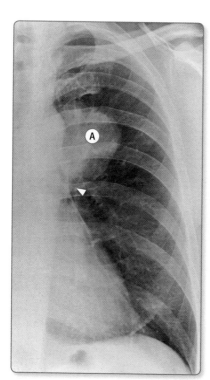

Figure 3.34 Chest X-ray showing pulmonary mass lesion (bronchogenic malignancy) (A) forming acute angles with the mediastinal surface (arrowhead).

sign indicates loss of a contour of a structure as a result of an adjacent abnormality (**Figure 3.36**).

Table 3.8 shows the differential diagnosis for a mediastinal mass.

Anterior mediastinal masses

Radiographic findings

Several findings are associated with anterior mediastinal masses (**Figure 3.37**). There is loss of visibility of the heart border on the affected side (the silhouette sign), with the superior vena cava obscured by right-sided masses. The trachea is deviated away from the affected side.

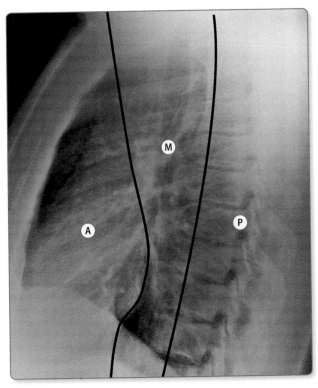

Figure 3.35 Lateral X-ray showing the division of the mediastinum into anterior (A), middle (M) and posterior (P) compartments to help develop differential diagnoses. Pathological conditions arise in structures in these compartments.

The heart border normally lies medial to the hilar vessels. Large anterior mediastinal masses may be difficult to distinguish from cardiac enlargement, except that the apparent heart border (i.e. the mass) overlies the hilum. This is the hilum overlay sign.

Middle mediastinal masses
Figures 3.38 show examples of middle mediastinal masses.

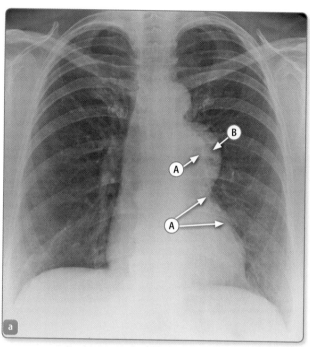

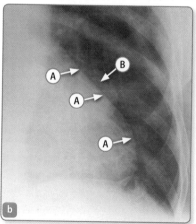

Figure 3.36 Chest X-rays illustrating the silhouette sign. (a) The left cardiac border (A) is indistinguishable from the large mass abutting it (B); the silhouette has been lost. (b) Preservation of the left cardiac border (A) indicates that the lesion (B) is not in contact with the heart and must lie in the lung parenchyma posteriorly.

Location of mass	Type of mass
Anterior	The four Ts, in order of frequency:
	• thymoma
	• terrible lymphoma (Figure 3.37)
	• teratoma
	• thyroid masses – rarely massive, more common at thoracic inlet
Middle	Lymphadenopathy (lymphoma, sarcoid or tuberculosis)
	Foregut duplication cysts (**Figure 3.38**): bronchogenic cysts or oesophageal duplications
	Oesophageal mass
Posterior	Neurogenic tumours (**Figure 3.39**), most commonly: • schwannomas and neurofibromas in adults • neuroblastomas and ganglioneuroblastomas in children
	Aneurysms of the descending aorta
	Lymphadenopathy
	Paraspinal abscesses
	Rarely, extramedullary haematopoiesis (e.g. thalassaemia)

Table 3.8 Differential diagnosis of mediastinal masses

Radiographic findings

Findings associated with middle mediastinal masses are splaying of the carina and disruption of the azygo-oesophageal line. Abnormal tissue is present in the aortopulmonary window.

Posterior mediastinal masses

Figure 3.39 shows an example of a posterior mediastinal mass.

Radiographic findings

A finding associated with posterior mediastinal masses is splaying or thinning of the posterior ribs. The silhouette sign is absent, i.e. the borders of the heart and aortic knuckle are visible.

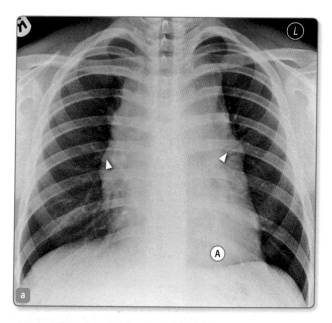

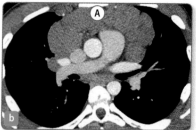

Figure 3.37 (a) Chest X-ray showing massive anterior mediastinal lymphadenopathy secondary to Hodgkin lymphoma. The superior vena cava and upper portion of the left heart border are not visible as separate from the mass (A). The hilar vessels (arrowheads) are visible medial to the boundaries of the mass bilaterally (the hilum overlay sign). (b) Computerised tomography scan of the same patient, showing extensive abnormal soft tissue (A) over the anterior surface of the mediastinum.

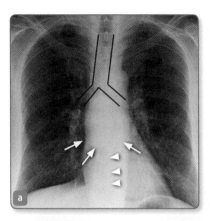

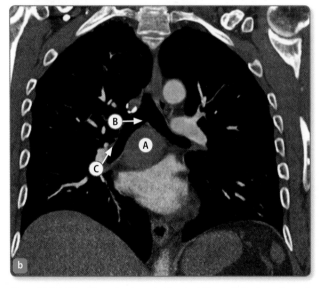

Figure 3.38 (a) Chest X-ray showing a significant middle mediastinal mass (arrows). The mass is visible but subtle and is splaying the carina (outlined) and disrupting the azygo-oesophageal line (arrowheads). (b) Coronal computerised tomography scan from just below the carina. The 5-cm soft tissue middle mediastinal mass (A) lies underneath the carina (B), distorting the bronchus intermedius (C).

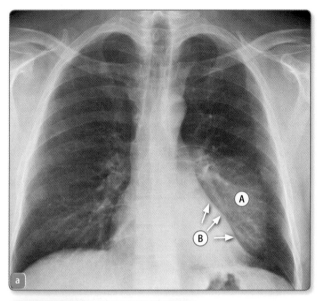

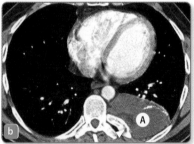

Figure 3.39 (a) Chest X-ray showing a large left posterior mediastinal mass (A) The partial hilum overlay sign shows the mass to be either anterior or posterior, but preservation of the left heart border (B) combined with slight sclerosis and modelling deformity of the left 8th rib, indicates that it is posterior. (b) Computerised tomography scan of the same patient, showing a large soft tissue mass in the left posterior mediastinum (A), with marginal calcification. A rib is distorted (arrowhead).

3.6 Diaphragm, subdiaphragmatic area and chest wall abnormalities

Diaphragm paralysis

Each side of the diaphragm is innervated by the phrenic nerve. Unilateral paralysis of a hemidiaphragm occurs if the phrenic nerve on that side is damaged. Damage often results from malignancy (e.g. from mediastinal adenopathy damaging the nerve) but can be from benign causes (e.g. after a viral illness).

The diaphragm on the affected side is elevated (**Figure 3.40**). To confirm weakness, direct observation under X-ray screening or ultrasound will show poor or even paradoxical movement. A CT scan is necessary if malignancy is suspected.

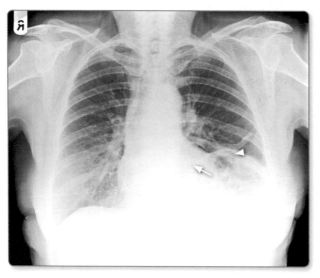

Figure 3.40 Chest X-ray showing elevated left hemidiaphragm (arrowhead). The condition was presumed to be caused by viral infection and improved spontaneously over 2 years.

Ruptured diaphragm

A ruptured hemidiaphragm usually occurs after major trauma. If significant amounts of abdominal organs herniate into the chest, the lungs or heart may be compressed. Also, the bowel may strangulate as it passes through the defect. Rupture is more common on the left side because the right may be protected by the underlying liver.

The affected diaphragm may be elevated, with loops of bowel visible in the chest. This finding may be mistaken for a raised diaphragm, and CT or magnetic resonance imaging may be necessary to show the defect in the diaphragm.

Pneumoperitoneum

A pneumoperitoneum appears on an erect chest X-ray as air below the diaphragm (**Figure 3.41**). It may not be visible on a supine

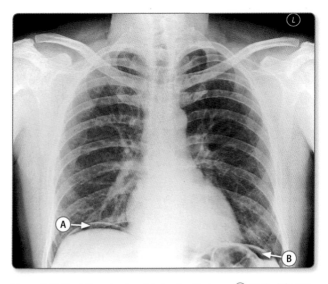

Figure 3.41 Chest X-ray showing air below the diaphragm Ⓐ. On the left, air is also around the bowel Ⓑ.

film because the air will pass to the most anterior part of the abdomen and not necessarily outline the diaphragm.

Pneumoperitoneum is normal after laparotomy or laparoscopic surgery, when residual peritoneal air is visible for a week or sometimes

Clinical insight

Herniation through a defect may not occur immediately. Some patients present with symptoms only years after the original event, sometimes with serious consequences. Bowel may necrose if strangulated as it passes through the defect.

more. At other times, pneumoperitoneum almost always signifies serious abdominal pathological changes caused by bowel perforation.

Rib fracture and metastasis

Isolated fractures are usually not clinically significant, except for causing considerable pain (**Figure 3.42**). However, ribs

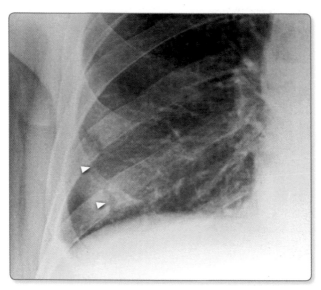

Figure 3.42 Chest X-ray showing mildly displaced rib fractures (arrowheads).

that are significantly displaced can injure adjacent pleura, lung or other adjacent structures (**Figure 3.43**). They may cause pneumothorax or haemothorax, pulmonary bleeding, splenic or liver lacerations (if the lower ribs are involved) and bleeding from the major branches of the aorta (if the upper ribs are involved). Multiple adjacent rib fractures causing flail chest can cause respiratory compromise because of poor ventilation of the affected hemithorax. Mechanical ventilation may be necessary.

Rib fractures may be difficult to see on a plain chest X-ray but pulmonary complications should be evident. A CT scan is

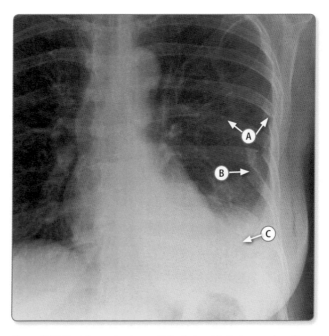

Figure 3.43 Chest X-rays showing multiple displaced rib fractures and small haemothorax. Slightly displaced rib fractures (A), very displaced rib fracture (B) and small left haemothorax (C).

needed urgently if concern exists about possible liver, splenic or aortic branch bleeding.

The ribs are common sites for metastases. Some primary malignancies, especially prostate, cause sclerotic lesions (areas of denser bone caused by sclerosis). However, most malignancies cause an area of lucency in the bone because of a destructive process and may have a soft tissue mass component (**Figure 3.44**). Pathological fractures are common because metastases usually weaken the bone.

Subcutaneous emphysema

Subcutaneous emphysema, also called surgical emphysema, is caused by air in the soft tissues of the chest wall (**Figure 3.45**). Air in the subcutaneous tissues of the skin passes along soft tissue planes and may be extensive. Subcutaneous emphysema is rarely dangerous in itself but its causes

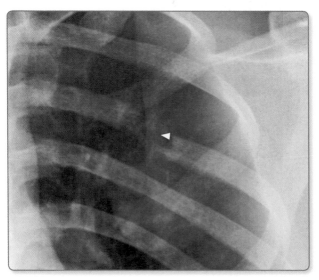

Figure 3.44 Chest X-ray with view of lytic metastasis in rib (arrowhead).

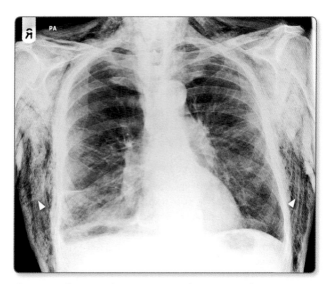

Figure 3.45 Chest X-ray showing extensive subcutaneous emphysema (arrowheads) all around the chest, originally caused by a pneumothorax.

may be. The condition is usually secondary to penetrating trauma, pneumothorax, pneumomediastinum or insertion of a chest drain. Subcutaneous emphysema may signify that a chest drain is blocked or not fully positioned in the chest.

Thoracic infections

4.1 Community-acquired pneumonia

Pneumonia is inflammation of the lungs that causes consolidation. It is usually caused by infection and can be unilateral or bilateral, and patchy lobar or diffuse.

Community-acquired pneumonia is infection of the lungs by bacteria or viruses. The most common pathogen is *Streptococcus pneumoniae* (pneumococcus); others include *Haemophilus influenzae*, *Legionella* species, mycoplasmas and respiratory viruses. Lobar pneumonia is unifocal, usually involving a single lobe, whereas bronchopneumonia is multifocal. The chest X-ray plays an important role in diagnosis and in assessing severity, complications and response to treatment.

Key facts
- Pneumococcus is the most common pathogen
- Consolidation is either lobar or patchy (bronchopneumonia)
- Chest X-ray is a key tool for diagnosis and management

Radiographic findings
Lobar consolidation appears as extensive opacification of part or whole of a lobe. An air bronchogram is often seen in the consolidation. The lobar pneumonia is often demarcated by a fissure; the horizontal fissure separates the opacification from the middle lobe (**Figure 4.1**).

Bronchopneumonia appears as patchy multifocal areas of consolidation (**Figure 4.2**). Complications may occur with cavitation, lung abscess or empyema. Cavitation appears as a lucency in the consolidation (**Figure 4.3**).

Management
Uncomplicated cases are most often treated with empirical antibiotics; organism-specific antibiotics are used once culture results are available. Most cases are followed up with repeat

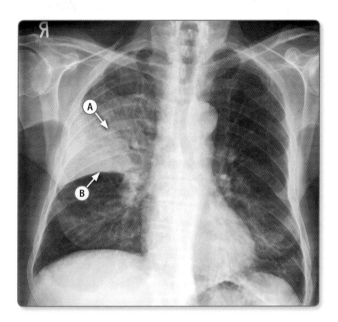

Figure 4.1 Chest X-ray showing infective consolidation in the right upper lobe (A), bounded inferiorly by the horizontal fissure (B), i.e. lobar pneumonia.

plain X-rays, and further imaging by computerised tomography (CT) is helpful in non-resolving pneumonia or to assess complications.

4.2 Active tuberculosis

Infection by *Mycobacterium tuberculosis* is the cause of tuberculosis and over 90% of mycobacteriinfections in humans. *M. avium* complex and *M. kansasii* are non-tuberculous opportunistic mycobacteria commonly responsible for pulmonary infection in humans.

Pulmonary tuberculosis spreads by droplet infection. The two patterns of active infection depend on recognition of hypersensitivity to the tuberculous protein.

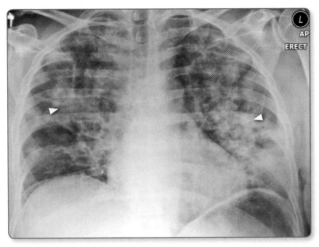

Figure 4.2 Chest X-ray showing patchy multifocal consolidation (arrowheads) in both lungs in bronchopneumonia.

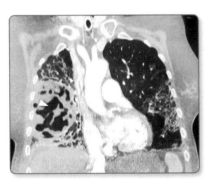

Figure 4.3 Reformatted coronal computerised tomography in pneumococcal pneumonia, showing large cavitating consolidation (arrowhead) on the right and patchy consolidation on the left.

Primary tuberculosis

This is usually seen in children not immunised with bacillus Calmette–Guérin (BCG) and is acquired from a contact by droplet infection. Adults not exposed to tuberculous bacteria or BCG may also develop primary tuberculosis. This type of tuberculosis usually manifests as pneumonic consolidation, adenopathy, miliary nodules or pleural effusion (usually not empyema).

Postprimary tuberculosis

Patients who are hypersensitive to the tuberculoprotein from past exposure tend to develop postprimary tuberculosis. This type of tuberculosis usually affects the apices or the apical segments of the lower lobes and appears as infiltrates, cavitation or empyema. Tuberculosis is increasingly seen in immuno-compromised or HIV-infected adults; pulmonary tuberculosis is common in patients with AIDS.

The characteristics of primary and postprimary tuberculosis overlap, particularly in immunocompromised patients. Therefore these conditions are dealt with under the common heading of *pulmonary tuberculosis* for the purposes of this book.

Tuberculous adenopathy

Tuberculous adenopathy is seen usually in children or young adults. The condition is always associated with infiltrates or consolidation in the adjacent lung. The adenopathy is usually unilateral and may involve hilar or mediastinal nodes (paratracheal nodes), or a combination of both. Bilateral hilar adenopathy is occasionally seen but is almost always asymmetrical. In children, the large nodes may compress the trachea or bronchi, leading to lobar or lung atelectasis. Adenopathy may rupture into adjacent bronchus and caseous material is discharged, causing endobronchial spread of tuberculosis. Rupture into a blood vessel causes haematogenous dissemination of disease, i.e. miliary tuberculosis.

Radiographic findings

Tuberculous adenopathy is typically unilateral, hilar or paratracheal (mediastinal) and appears as an enlarged hilum or widening of the mediastinum (**Figure 4.4a**). The adenopathy has an asymmetrical, matted appearance with loss of outline and forms a confluent soft tissue mass. Rarely, bilateral hilar enlargement is present but asymmetrical. On CT, nodes show central low density or caseation (**Figure 4.4b**).

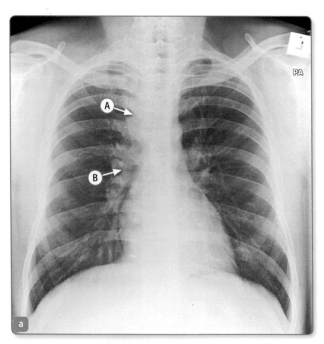

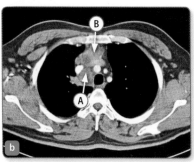

Figure 4.4 (a) Chest X-ray showing features of tuberculous mediastinal adenopathy: widening of the superior mediastinum (A) and hilar adenopathy (B) with enlarged right hilum. (b) Axial computerised tomography scan of the same patient, showing right paratracheal (A) and anterior mediastinal matted adenopathy with central low density, i.e. caseation in the anterior mediastinal nodes (B).

Tuberculous pleural effusion and empyema

Tuberculous pleural effusion is often seen in primary tuberculosis and presents as large unilateral effusion. Other signs of adenopathy or lung infiltrates may be present. The condition usually resolves after treatment, without residual scarring or calcification. However, the pleural effusion in postprimary tuberculosis is inevitably an empyema, which tends to heal with pleural calcification and scarring.

Radiographic findings

A large unilateral pleural effusion is apparent. Simple effusion and empyema have similar features on plain X-ray (**Figure 4.5**). CT may show pleural thickening or loculation in empyema.

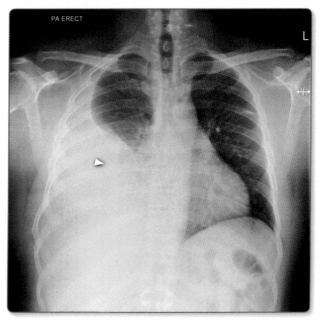

Figure 4.5 Chest X-ray showing large right pleural effusion (arrowhead) with mediastinal shift to the left.

Miliary tuberculosis

Miliary tuberculosis is a consequence of haematogenous spread of tuberculosis by rupture of tuberculous granulomas or caseous material into the bloodstream. The resulting widespread dissemination occurs in both primary and postprimary tuberculosis. Miliary tuberculosis appears on chest X-rays and CT scans as widespread fine (miliary) nodules of 1–2 mm (**Figure 4.6**). The patient is often acutely unwell, but the nodules clear completely with treatment and leave no residual features on X-ray.

Tuberculous infiltrates, endobronchial tuberculosis and tuberculous cavities

Consolidation, infiltrates and endobronchial spread of tuberculosis are seen in primary and postprimary tuberculosis. Cavitation is almost entirely seen in postprimary tuberculosis. Lesions involve the apices of the lungs or the apical segments of the lower lobes in over 90% of cases. Cavitation is seen in over half of cases, usually leading to fibrosis and scarring. Cavities are thick-walled and develop insidiously (**Figure 4.7**). Scarring leads to loss of volume and architectural distortion.

Endobronchial spread of tuberculosis occurs because of bronchial dissemination. It appears as widespread patchy consolidation (bronchopneumonia) and a tree-in-bud appearance involving the bronchioles (**Figure 4.8**).

Management

An antituberculous regimen is key to successful treatment. Corticosteroid drugs combined with antituberculous drugs may be used to treat tuberculosis involving the pleura, pericardium or meninges.

4.3 Old tuberculosis

Patients who have had pulmonary tuberculosis may have residual radiological signs of old and inactive tuberculosis. These signs are calcified nodes in the mediastinum and hila secondary to tuberculous adenopathy or a healed calcified primary focus in the lung parenchyma. Other radiological features include

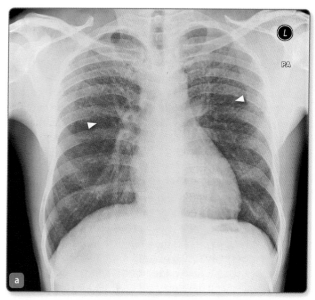

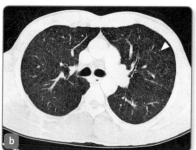

Figure 4.6 Chest X-ray (a) and axial computerised tomography (b) in miliary tuberculosis, showing widespread fine nodules (arrowheads) in both lungs.

scarring in the apices, with loss of volume, bronchiectasis, cysts and destroyed lung. Old cavities may be present in the apices. Complications of old tuberculosis include aspergilloma in the cavities (see section 4.5, p. 123). Old tuberculous empyema often appears as dense and coarse pleural calcification in a hemithorax, often encasing the lung.

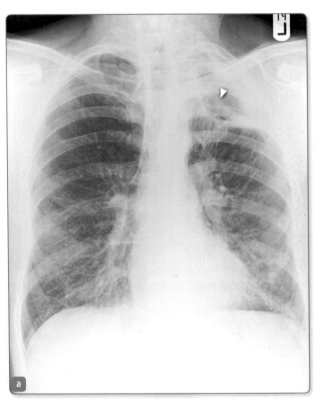

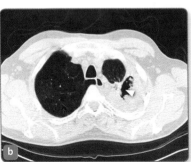

Figure 4.7 (a) Chest X-ray of tuberculosis cavity (arrowhead) in the left apex, with irregular thick wall and scarring. (b) Axial computerised tomography scan of tuberculosis cavity (arrowhead), from the same patient.

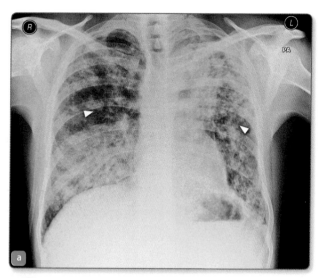

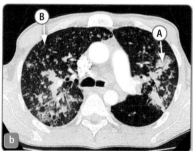

Figure 4.8 (a) Chest X-ray of tuberculous bronchopneumonia, showing widespread patchy areas of consolidation (arrowheads) in both lungs. (b) Axial computerised tomography scan of endobronchial tuberculosis, with patchy peribronchial opacities (A) and bronchiolar involvement, i.e. tree-in-bud appearance (B).

The chest X-rays and CT scans in **Figures 4.9** and **4.10** show the various radiological features of old tuberculosis. Calcified nodes and calcified tuberculous granulomas are present, with scarring and loss of volume of the apices. Destroyed parenchyma in the apices is replaced by severely dilated bronchi. Thickening of apical pleura is associated with old tuberculosis.

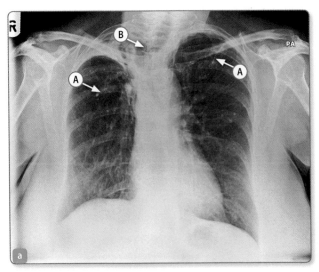

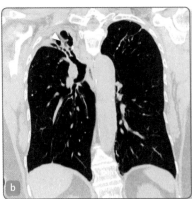

Figure 4.9 (a) Chest X-ray of old tuberculosis, showing old healed calcified granulomas (A) in both lungs and nodes. Also visible is right apical fibrosis, with loss of volume, tracheal deviation (B) and elevation of the right hilum. (b) Coronal reformatted computerised tomography scan of the same patient. Right apical scarring shows bronchiectasis (arrowhead). Calcified mediastinal nodes are present.

Old tuberculosis empyema

Old tuberculous empyema presents as extensive coarse and diffuse pleural calcification. The calcification is usually unilateral, with loss of volume and encasement of the lung (**Figure 4.11**).

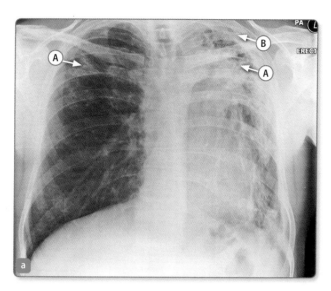

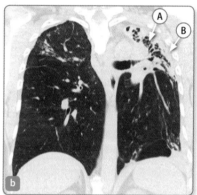

Figure 4.10 Chest X-ray (a) and computerised tomography (b) images of bilateral apical fibrosis Ⓐ in old tuberculosis, more on the left, with left apical pleural thickening Ⓑ.

Radiological evidence of surgical treatment in tuberculosis

Before antituberculous drugs were introduced, pulmonary tuberculosis was treated surgically. Treatment included surgical

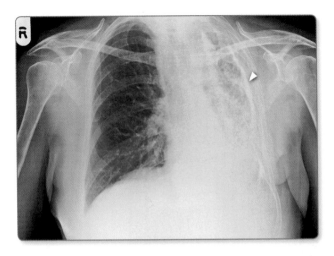

Figure 4.11 Chest X-ray of old tuberculosis empyema on the left, with extensive pleural calcification (arrowhead) and loss of volume of the hemithorax.

atelectasis of the affected lobes of the lung by thoracoplasty or plombage. These procedures are now rare.

Thoracoplasty involved resection of parts of ribs, with atelectasis of the underlying infected lobe or drainage of empyema. Evidence of thoracoplasty appears on X-rays as marked deformity of the hemithorax.

Plombage

Plombage involved inserting various inert materials extrapleurally to cause atelectasis of the infected lung. These materials included paraffin wax, air, plastic foam or sponge (**Figures 4.12 and 4.13**), Lucite balls (**Figure 4.14**) and oil. Late complications of these procedures include leakage of plombage material, fistulae formation and late infection .

4.4 *Pneumocystis* pneumonia

Pneumocystis pneumonia is caused by the opportunistic fungal pathogen *Pneumocystis jiroveci* (formerly known as

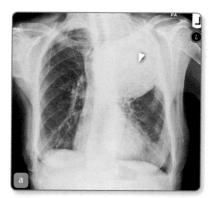

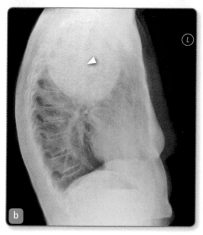

Figure 4.12 Frontal (a) and lateral (b) chest X-rays of plombage in the left apex. Fine lucencies caused by air pockets are seen in the sponge (arrowheads). Evidence of partial rib resection is present, and calcification and scarring around the margin of the plombage is visible.

P. carinii). *Pneumocystis* pneumonia is a common cause of morbidity and mortality in HIV-infected or otherwise immunocompromised patients. Onset is insidious, with malaise, dyspnoea, non-productive cough and weight loss. *Pneumocystis* pneumonia is still considered an AIDS-defining infection in HIV-infected patients, whose low CD4 lymphocyte count predisposes them to *Pneumocystis* infection.

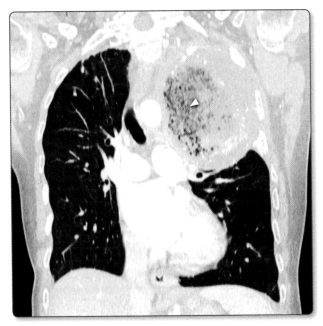

Figure 4.13 Coronal reformatted computerised tomography scan of the same patient as in Figure 4.12, showing fine lucencies in the sponge plombage (arrowhead).

Key facts

- Opportunistic infection by *P. jiroveci*.
- Seen in patients with HIV infection or otherwise compromised immune system.
- Typically seen on imaging as symmetrical diffuse interstitial infiltration of the lungs.

Radiographic findings

Typically, diffuse, symmetrical interstitial 'ground glass' infiltrates are present in the lungs, with fine reticular opacification (**Figure 4.15**). Perihilar distribution of the infiltrates is characteristic, with sparing of apices. Air bronchograms are present.

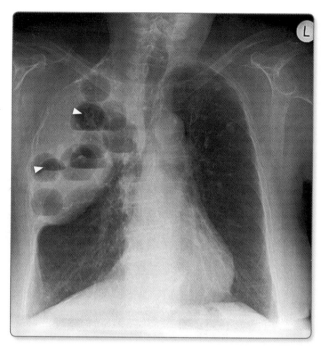

Figure 4.14 Chest X-ray showing surgical plombage treatment of tuberculosis with Lucite balls (arrowheads), seen as multiple thin-walled balls in the right upper lobe. Several of these balls contain air–fluid levels, usually caused by infection.

Diffuse ground glass opacification is visible on CT, and the air bronchograms appear as dark or black bronchi on a background of diffuse opacification; this is the black bronchus sign (**Figure 4.16**). Atypical imaging features include focal areas of infiltration, nodular opacities and occasionally cavitation or pneumatocoeles. Pleural effusions and adenopathy are rare.

Management

Diagnosis is usually suspected in an appropriate setting and based on combined clinical and imaging features. However,

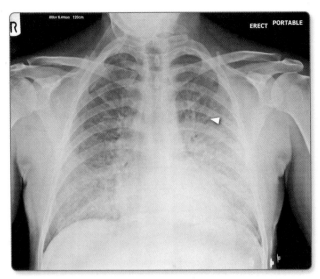

Figure 4.15 Chest X-ray showing diffuse opacification in the lungs (arrowhead) with sparing of the apices and air bronchograms in a patient with *Pneumocystis* pneumonia.

bronchoscopy with bronchoalveolar lavage is the gold standard for diagnosing *Pneumocystis* pneumonia. *P. jiroveci* cannot be cultured but tests for biomedical markers, including polymerase chain reaction to detect *P. jiroveci* DNA, may be useful.

Trimethoprim–sulfamethoxazole is used for prophylaxis and first-line treatment of *Pneumocystis* pneumonia. Adjuvant corticosteroid therapy is also used.

4.5 Fungal infection: aspergilloma

Several species of fungi can infect the lungs. Fungal infections are seen mainly in HIV-infected or otherwise immunocompromised patients. The commonest fungal infection of the lungs is *Aspergillus*; the main causative organism is *A. fumigatus*. Three main patterns of fungal infection of the lung are recognised.

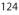

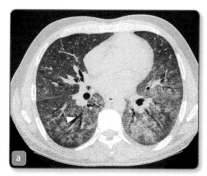

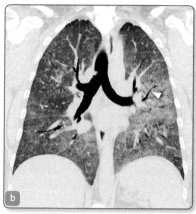

Figure 4.16 Axial (a) and coronal reformatted (b) computerised tomography scans of the same patient as in Figure 4.15, showing extensive ground glass opacification and fine reticular opacification. The bronchi (arrowheads) appear as black on a background opacification (the black bronchus sign).

- Aspergilloma (fungal ball) is the saprophytic colonisation of a preexisting cavity.
- Invasive pulmonary aspergillosis is radiologically indistinguishable from other causes of consolidation, is seen in immunocompromised patients and is associated with high morbidity and mortality.
- Allergic bronchopulmonary aspergillosis is caused by a hypersensitivity reaction to the pathogen and is dealt with in section 9.2.

Aspergilloma

Aspergilloma, also known as mycetoma, is caused by sapro-phytic colonisation of a preexisting lung cavity by *Aspergillus*. The *Aspergillus* hyphae mat to form a fungal ball. Aspergillomas are commonly seen in cavities caused by previous tuberculosis, large emphysematous bullae, pulmonary infarcts, sarcoid, bron-chiectasis and carcinoma. They tend to occur in the apices or in the apical segment of the lower lobes; these areas are typical sites for tuberculous cavities and bullae.

Aspergillomas are mostly asymptomatic but may present with haemoptysis. They have distinctive features on X-ray, and most are diagnosed by analysing chest X-rays. The differential diagnosis includes mobile blood clot in a cavity, intracavitary tumour and hydatid cyst.

Key facts

- Aspergillomas are fungal balls.
- They occur in preexisting cavities, usually those secondary to tuberculosis.
- On chest X-ray, an aspergilloma appears as a well-defined intracavitary mass, mainly in the upper zones; a crescent sign is typical.
- Aspergillomas are asymptomatic but occasionally present with haemoptysis.

Radiographic findings

An aspergilloma appears as a well-defined mass with smooth outline in a cavity, commonly in the upper zones. A typical finding is a crescent of air between the smooth mass and the wall of the cavity: the air crescent sign (**Figure 4.17**). The fungal ball is usually mobile in the cavity, and X-rays obtained with a change of patient position (i.e. lateral decubitus or supine views) often show the intracavitary mass and air crescent in dif-ferent positions. The mass may infrequently be fixed to the wall of the cavity, secondary to either inflammation or carcinoma. Fluid level may be seen, but calcification is extremely rare.

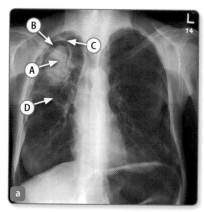

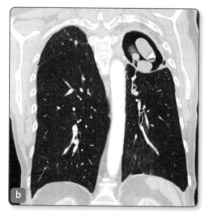

Figure 4.17 (a) Chest X-ray showing a cavity in the right upper lobe with a smoothly outlined oval mass: aspergilloma (A) in a dependent position. The air crescent sign (B) is a curvilinear lucency around the upper and lateral margins of the mass; the wall of the cavity (C) is mostly thin but with some thickening inferomedially. Some volume has been lost from the right upper lobe, and the horizontal fissure is displaced upwards (D). (b) Reformatted coronal computerised tomography scan in another patient, showing three smooth oval intracavitary masses in a left apical cavity (arrowhead).

Management

Aspergillomas are often diagnosed by analysing a plain chest X-ray or CT scan. Serum precipitins for *Aspergillus* confirm the diagnosis. Severe hemoptysis, if present, is often treated with bronchial artery embolisation or surgery. Biopsy may be done if concern exists about a malignancy and allows appropriate treatment.

Interstitial lung diseases

chapter
5

Many types of interstitial lung disease exist. Some (e.g. asbestosis and silicosis) are also termed pneumoconioses and are caused by occupational exposure to harmful particles. Many are rare, and frequently the plain chest X-ray is not helpful. High-resolution computerised tomography (CT) of the chest is invaluable in assessing such patients.

This chapter discusses four interstitial lung diseases. They are the more common diseases and have discriminating features on X-rays.

5.1 Sarcoidosis

Sarcoidosis is a systemic disease characterised by the presence of non-caseating epithelioid cell granulomas. organs and can resolve spontaneously or lead to severe chronic ill health or death.

Sarcoidosis is common in North European countries (5–25 cases/100 000 persons). It is often asymptomatic and may be underdiagnosed in some countries, depending on the level of health care available. Many features of the disease can mimic cancer or chronic infections such as tuberculosis.

Key facts
- Typical age at presentation is 20–40 years.
- Systemic symptoms (e.g. fever, weight loss, lethargy and joint pain) are common initially.
- The skin condition erythema nodosum may be present.
- Respiratory symptoms may include cough and shortness of breath.

Radiographic findings
The typical chest X-ray findings are caused by mediastinal

> **Clinical insight**
>
> Sarcoidosis chest disease is often found incidentally, even in patients without respiratory symptoms. Its presence can play a key role in making the diagnosis.

lymphadenopathy and granulomas in the lung parenchyma. Sarcoid can be staged according to the chest X-ray appearance (**Table 5.1**). Most patients present with stage 1 or 2 disease. The lower the stage at presentation, the greater the chance of resolution of symptoms and signs on X-ray.

Adenopathy is common at presentation but will usually disappear or greatly reduce during the course of the disease. The commonest combinations are of bilateral hilar, paratracheal and aortopulmonary adenopathy. They are usually visible on chest X-ray (**Figure 5.1**) but, if suspected, better shown on chest CT (**Figure 5.2a**). Only one or two of these types of adenopathy may be visible, which often raises the possibility of alternative diagnoses (e.g. lymphoma or cancer). The incidence of calcification is high (20% over 10 years) if nodes persist during the disease.

Fewer than half of patients have parenchymal changes at diagnosis. A wide range of abnormalities are possible. The commonest finding is multiple small irregular nodules of 1–5 mm lying bilaterally in the mid and upper zones. These nodules may coalesce into larger opacities, which can cavitate. The pattern of nodules follows the distribution of lymphatic channels; this is more evident on CT than on X-rays (**Figure 5.3**). Imaging shows beading of bronchovascular bundles, irregularity of fissures and subpleural nodules, with thickening of interlobular septa caused by diffuse thickening of the lymphatic vessels (**Figure 5.2b**).

Stage	Description
0	Normal X-ray
1	Nodal enlargement only
2	Nodal enlargement and parenchymal disease
3	Parenchymal opacity without adenopathy or evidence of fibrosis
4	Lung fibrosis (distortion, volume loss and cysts)

Table 5.1 Staging sarcoid

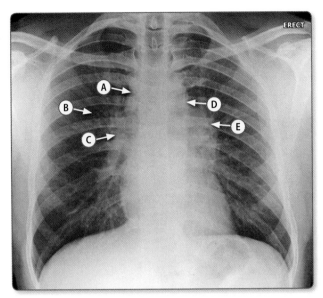

Figure 5.1 Chest X-ray showing sarcoidosis: mediastinal and hilar adenopathy. Ⓐ Right paratracheal adenopathy. Ⓑ A few small parenchymal nodules. Ⓒ Right hilar adenopathy. Ⓓ Aortopulmonary window adenopathy. Ⓔ Left hilar adenopathy.

Fibrosis is evident in 5–25% of patients at presentation. It will develop in 10–15% of patients presenting with stage 0–2 disease over 2–15 years. Fibrosis consists of coarse linear shadows radiating from hilar into mid and upper zones, with retraction and distortion of parenchyma. Marked traction bronchial dilatation may be present. There may be honey-combing, cyst formation and cor pulmonale in end-stage disease.

Diagnosis can be made on the CT findings if they are typical and associated with the usual pattern of adenopathy. However, take care to avoid mistaking the other main differential diagnoses: lymphangitis, carcinomatosis and tuberculosis. If doubt exists, take biopsies of nodes or lung parenchyma.

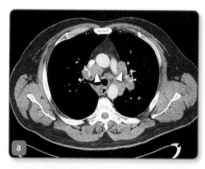

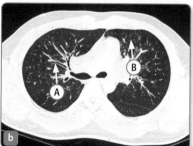

Figure 5.2 Computerised tomography scans showing sarcoid. (a) Extensive mediastinal adenopathy - vascular structures are dense because of intravenous contrast (arrowheads). The lighter grey tissues are enlarged lymph nodes. (b) (A) Thickening and nodularity of bronchovascular bundles. (B) Fine nodules in parenchyma of the upper zones. This combination is characteristic of sarcoid.

Management

Treatment is based on oral corticosteroids in cases of progressive or symptomatic stage 2 or 3 disease. Short-term use of oral corticosteroids benefits many patients but long-term use is controversial. Other immunosuppressive agents may be used.

5.2 Usual interstitial pneumonia

Usual interstitial pneumonia is the most common of a group of inflammatory and fibrotic lung diseases termed the idiopathic interstitial pneumonias. Usual interstitial pneumonia is the histological description of the disease; the associated clinical syndrome is idiopathic pulmonary fibrosis (previously called cryptogenic fibrosing alveolitis).

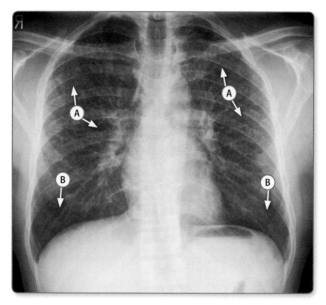

Figure 5.3 Chest X-ray showing parenchymal sarcoidosis. (A) Bilateral upper zone nodularity, particularly along the bronchovascular bundles. (B) Sparing of the lower zones. Vascularity essentially appears normal.

Key facts

- Usual interstitial pneumonia has an insidious onset of cough and breathlessness, sometimes with systemic features. It is more common in males, and most patients are over 50 years old at presentation.

- Prognosis is poor. Mean survival after diagnosis is 2–9 years. Death usually results from respiratory failure or secondary cardiovascular disease, but there is also an increased incidence of lung malignancy.

Clinical insight

Usual interstitial pneumonia is by definition idiopathic, but a nearly identical radiological and pathological pattern can be seen in patients who have developed fibrosis secondary to some connective tissue disorders or heavy asbestos exposure.

- Lung function tests show a restrictive pattern.
- Pathologically, there is a patchy and variable distribution of areas of fibrosis of different stages of maturity. Normal areas may be interspersed with areas of severe fibrosis. Fibrosis causes architectural distortion and a honeycomb pattern of scarring.

Radiographic findings

Most patients will have an abnormal chest X-ray, but the abnormalities are often subtle. It is important to also obtain high-resolution CT scans and lung function tests if the diagnosis is suspected.

The classic findings on X-ray (**Figure 5.4**) are a basally predominant, peripheral subpleural distribution of reticular

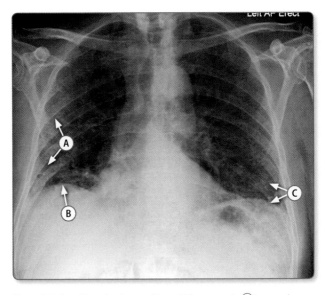

Figure 5.4 Chest X-ray showing usual interstitial pneumonia. Ⓐ Increased shadowing in the periphery of the lungs, worse towards the bases. Ⓑ Reduced lung volumes (raised diaphragm). Ⓒ Fine nodularity increasing peripheral density.

nodular shadowing. The shadowing may just be a vague increased peripheral density early in the disease course. As the disease progresses, lung volumes shrink and the shadowing becomes coarser and more honeycomb.

Honeycomb cysts may rupture to cause a pneumomediastinum (**Figure 5.5**) or pneumothorax. Other complications include infection, often with opportunistic organisms and lung cancer (usual interstitial pneumonia increases the risk fivefold).

High-resolution CT is important in making the diagnosis. Lung biopsy is not indicated if high-resolution CT scans have the classic appearance of usual interstitial pneumonia. The characteristic features are peripheral reticulation or honeycombing with areas of traction bronchiectasis (**Figure 5.5**).

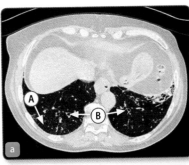
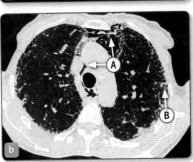

Figure 5.5 High-resolution computerised tomography scans showing usual interstitial pneumonia. (a) (**A**) Peripheral interstitial shadowing: early reticulation. (**B**) Traction bronchial ilatation. (b) A different patient with usual interstitial pneumonia has (**A**) a pneumomediastinum and (**B**) peripheral reticulation and early honeycombing.

Management

Treatment options are of limited benefit. Steroids and immuno-suppression are often tried, despite minimal evidence for their efficacy. Newer agents are being evaluated.

5.3 Asbestosis

Asbestosis is the fibrosing lung condition caused by exposure to asbestos fibres. It develops after a latent period of 20–40 years, and a large fibre load is needed to cause it. The most fibrogenic form of asbestos is crocidolite.

Patients present with cough and progressive breathlessness, although asbestosis progresses more slowly than usual inter-stitial pneumonia. Lung function tests again show a restrictive pattern.

Key facts

- The histological features of asbestosis are identical to those of usual interstitial pneumonia.
- Diagnosis is made on a combination of occupational history (including the amount and duration of expo-sure), radiographic findings, clinical features and lung function.
- Exposure to asbestos increases the risk of lung malignancy. Other complications of asbestos exposure are diffuse pleural thickening and mesothelioma. Pleural plaques are asymptomatic.

Radiographic findings

The chest X-ray is often normal when symptoms begin, and high-resolution CT changes are mild. If changes are visible on X-ray, the X-ray shows a pattern of abnormalities similar to those of usual interstitial pneumonia, although in most people asbestos plaques will also be present (**Figure 5.6**). The plaques are often calcified and therefore dense. The plaques appear as sheets of dense calcification if seen end on on the lateral chest wall or over the diaphragm. If viewed frontally, they are often described as shaped like a holly leaf.

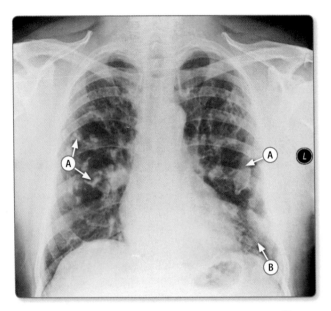

Figure 5.6 Chest X-ray showing asbestos plaques and mild asbestosis. (A) Calcified plaques. (B) Fine basal reticulonodularity caused by early asbestosis.

Basally predominant subpleural lines and dots and linear fibrotic lines are present on high-resolution CT (**Figure 5.7**) in early disease. The later changes are coarser than in usual interstitial pneumonia.

Management
No treatment is effective. In many countries, where for many years laws have prevented companies from exposing workers to asbestos, patients may be entitled to financial compensation through the courts.

5.4 Silicosis

Inhalation of free silica (silicon dioxide) particles can cause various pulmonary complications:

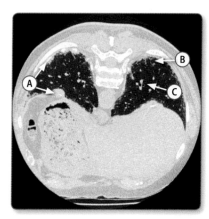

Figure 5.7 High-resolution computerised tomography scan showing asbestosis. (A) Calcified and non-calcified plaques. (B) Subpleural basal interstitial opacities and early reticulation. (B) Traction bronchiectasis.

- simple silicosis
- progressive massive fibrosis (conglomeration of nodules in the upper lobes, with peripheral emphysema)
- acute silicosis (after acute large exposure)
- chronic bronchitis
- emphysema
- tuberculosis
- lung cancer.

Silica inhalation is prevented by wearing appropriate respiratory protective masks. Silica dust is produced particularly during mining, sandblasting and ceramic manufacture.

Key facts

- Clinical features depend on the type of disease triggered in the patient. They also depend on the level and duration of exposure. In silicosis or progressive massive fibrosis, patients usually present with increasing breathlessness.
- Silica particles are toxic to macrophages and trigger formation of hyalinised nodules. This in turn leads to a fibrotic reaction that causes nodules to coalesce form the masses seen in progressive massive fibrosis. These are the main processes

seen on imaging. Air is also trapped in peripheral areas of the lungs.

Radiographic findings

The characteristic finding in early silicosis is multiple well-defined nodules of 1-3 mm predominantly in the

> ### Clinical insight
>
> If the disease progresses to progressive massive fibrosis, the nodules enlarge into peripheral upper zone masses, which can cavitate. The patient is usually experiencing breathlessness by this time. The masses are often bilateral but if unilateral can mimic cancer.

mid and upper zones of the lungs. Evidence of volume loss in the upper lobes may be present if the disease progresses to fibrosis (**Figure 5.8**). The nodules may calcify and are more apparent on CT (**Figure 5.9**). Air trapping may be visible elsewhere.

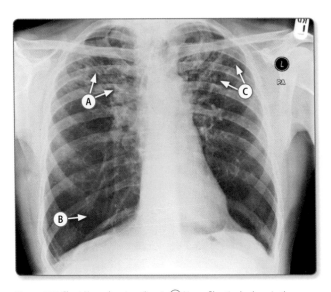

Figure 5.8 Chest X-ray showing silicosis. Ⓐ Linear fibrotic shadows in the upper zones, with elevated hila. Ⓑ Air trapping and emphysema in the lower zones. Ⓒ Small, well-defined, dense upper zone nodules.

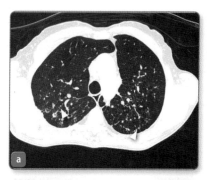

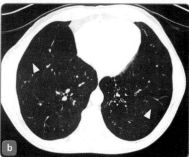

Figure 5.9 High-resolution computerised tomography scan showing silicosis. (a) Posterior lung nodules in the upper zone (arrowheads). (b) Air-trapping and emphysema in the lower zones (arrowheads).

Management

Management of silicosis comprises symptomatic relief and treatment of associated diseases (e.g. airway disease).

Bronchogenic malignancy and metastatic disease

Lung cancer is the most common cause of cancer-related death in the UK. When identified early, non–small-cell carcinoma may be resected, with survival rates of 40–85%. However, lung cancers more commonly present late and have a 5-year survival of around 10%.

Many lung cancers are first identified on chest X-ray. Chest X-ray is less sensitive than computerised tomography (CT) but remains a core diagnostic test. Identification of a nodule or mass on a chest X-ray in an adult should always raise the possibility of either primary or secondary malignancy. Review of old X-rays is invaluable in this context; nodules or masses that have not grown over 2 years are unlikely to be malignant. Correlation with the history and subsequent imaging tests (e.g. CT and positron emission tomography–CT) will help characterise and stage the malignancy.

This chapter presents a range of appearances of bronchogenic malignancy as well as metastatic pulmonary disease.

6.1 Bronchogenic malignancy

Hilar masses

Masses in the hilar regions (**Figure 6.1**) can easily be overlooked. A clear understanding of normal anatomy is vital for interpreting this complex region of the chest X-ray.

Key facts

- Compare the hilar points; a dense hilum suggests bronchogenic malignancy even if the contour of the hilum is normal. Loss of the normal concavity of the hilum usually indicates the presence of abnormal soft tissue.
- Hilar abnormalities are not necessarily caused by bronchogenic malignancy.

Clinical insight

Actively evaluate the hilar points and beware the dense hilum.

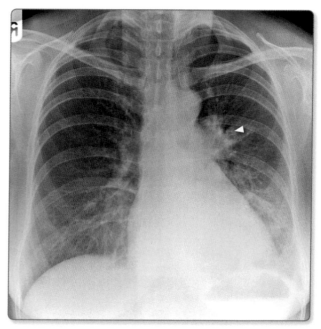

Figure 6.1 Posteroanterior chest X-ray showing a left hilar mass (arrowhead). The left hilum is denser than the right and the normal concavity of the hilar point has been lost, indicating the presence of abnormal tissue. The diagnosis is bronchogenic malignancy.

They may result from pathological nodal enlargement (e.g. lymphoma, tuberculosis and sarcoidosis) or vascular anomalies.

Radiographic findings

Increased hilar density and infilling of the normal hilar concavity may indicate the presence of smaller lesions. Large masses are usually obvious.

Management

Hilar abnormalities should be investigated by CT scanning.

Pancoast tumours

A Pancoast or superior sulcus tumour is a mass growing at the thoracic inlet. Symptoms are caused by the tumour directly invading the apical chest wall (**Figure 6.2**). These tumours classically cause Pancoast syndrome, which involves pain in the shoulder and along the ulnar nerve distribution of the arm and hand. Horner syndrome may also occur if there is invasion of the sympathetic chain.

> **Clinical insight**
>
> In Horner syndrome, compression of the cervical sympathetic nerve causes ipsilateral ptosis, miosis, enophthalmos and anhidrosis.

Key facts

- The superior sulcus is an uncommon location for bronchogenic malignancy (1–3% of all lung cancers).

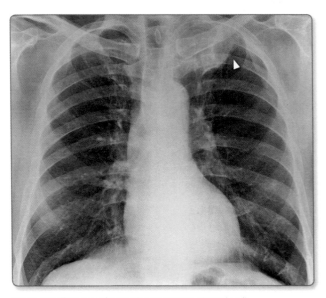

Figure 6.2 Chest X-ray showing Pancoast tumour (arrowhead).

- Pancoast tumours are rarely small cell in origin.
- Initial chest X-rays may not show abnormality if the tumour is small.

Radiographic findings

Chest X-ray shows opacification of the apex of the lung. Look for evidence of local bony destruction.

Management

Pancoast tumours are by definition stage T3 in the tumour, lymph node and metastasis (TNM) system. Surgery is indicated in patients who have very localised early disease. Irradiation may be used to palliate symptoms of pain in patients with unresectable disease.

Obstructive lesions

Lobar or total lung atelectasis on a chest X-ray (**Figure 6.3**) from an adult patient indicates a proximal bronchial obstruction. Unless the history clearly indicates foreign body inhalation or copious mucus production, endobronchial malignancy is the commonest cause and may be primary or secondary.

Key fact

- Patients with endobronchial pathological changes commonly have haemoptysis.

Radiographic findings

Radiographic signs of lobar or lung atelectasis (see section 3.2) may be the only sign of true endobronchial lesions. Large central lesions invading and obstructing the bronchus are usually visible as a mass.

Clinical insight

Lobar or lung atelectasis should prompt CT scanning and bronchoscopy if clinically appropriate.

Management

Management depends on cancer stage and tissue type.

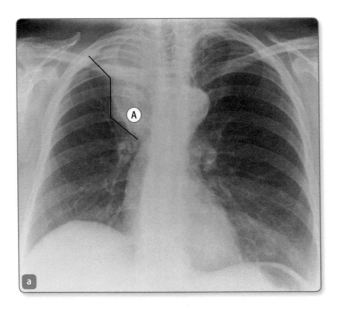

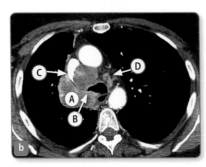

Figure 6.3 (a) Chest X-ray showing a right hilar mass (A) resulting in atelectasis of the right upper lobe. The inferior border of the atelectatic lobe and mass forms a sigmoid shape, the so-called Golden S sign, which characterises malignancy. (b) Axial computerised tomography scan from the same patient, showing the right hilar mass (A) and obliteration of the right upper lobe bronchus (B). The superior vena cava (C) is slightly compressed. Lymph nodes are visible in the subaortic fossa (D).

All cancer should ideally be managed in a multidisciplinary oncological setting.

Bronchoalveolar cell carcinoma

Bronchoalveolar cell carcinoma is a distinct subtype of adenocarcinoma that classically manifests as interstitial lung pathology on chest X-ray (**Figure 6.4**).

Key facts

- Bronchoalveolar carcinoma arises from type 2 pneumocytes and grows along alveolar septa.
- It may occur in non-smokers, e.g. complicating pulmonary fibrosis.

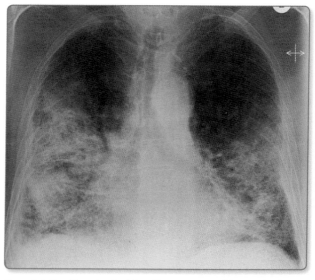

Figure 6.4 Chest X-ray showing bilateral lower zone consolidation in the absence of signs of infection, proved histologically to be multifocal bronchoalveolar cell carcinoma. The patient had a history of pulmonary fibrosis, a risk factor for malignancy.

Radiographic findings

Bronchoalveolar cell carcinoma may present as a solitary peripheral nodule, as multifocal consolidation (25% of cases) or in a rapidly progressing pneumonic pattern.

Management

Management depends on cancer stage and tissue type. All cancer should ideally be managed in a multidisciplinary oncological setting.

6.2 Metastatic disease

Lung metastases

The most common primary malignancies to metastasise to the lungs are cancers of the breast, colon, kidney, uterus, and head and neck. Some tumours have a particular predilection but are rare, e.g. choriocarcinoma, sarcomas, testicular tumours, thyroid tumours and melanoma. The plain chest X-ray is the most important initial investigation to show metastases (**Figure 6.5**), but CT is more accurate.

Radiographic findings

Metastases are generally rounded, well-defined nodules of varying sizes. They are usually of soft tissue density (**Figure 6.5**), unless they are from a carcinoma, which tends to calcify (e.g. osteosarcomas and mucin-producing adenocarcinomas of the colon). Calcification can also follow successful therapy. Metastases may be of soft, ground glass density and more difficult to identify, except on CT (**Figures 6.6 and 6.7**). Some may cavitate, especially if growing rapidly

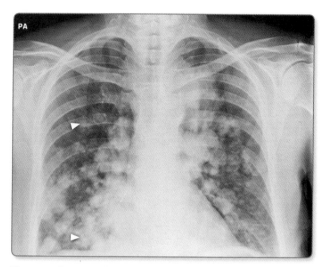

Figure 6.5 Chest X-ray showing multiple metastases: multiple rounded nodules of varying sizes throughout the lungs (arrowheads).

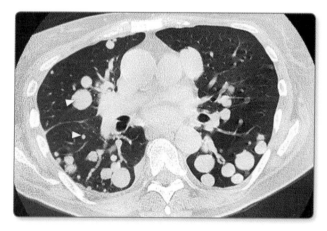

Figure 6.6 Computerised tomography scan showing lung metastases. Rounded soft tissue density nodules in both lungs (arrowheads).

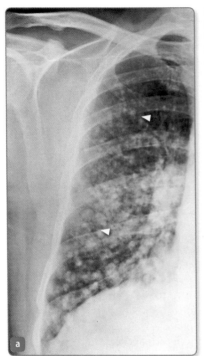

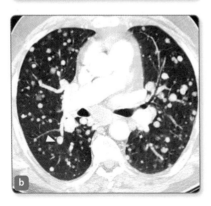

Figure 6.7 (a) Chest X-ray and (b) computerised tomography scan showing multiple small thyroid metastatic nodules (arrowheads).

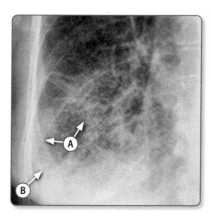

Figure 6.8 Chest X-ray showing lymphangitis. (A) Fine reticulonodular opacities, (B) small effusion.

with central necrosis. Peripheral metastases can occasionally cause a pneumothorax. The chest X-ray may also show signs of mediastinal adenopathy.

Lymphangitis carcinomatosa

Lymphangitis (**Figure 6.8**) is caused by malignant cells spreading through pulmonary lymphatic vessels. It most frequently arises from carcinomas of lung, breast, pancreas, stomach and colon.

Radiographic findings

Characteristic findings on chest X-ray are fine reticulonodular opacities with peripheral septal lines. Some patients have evidence of hilar adenopathy and small pleural effusions.

The changes are often unilateral or focal. If they are generalised, the main differential diagnosis is pulmonary oedema. CT (**Figure 6.9**) helps differentiate between the two conditions. Lymphangitis causes septal thickening that is often more nodular and pronounced than seen in oedema, and it persists despite diuretic therapy.

Endobronchial metastases

Tumours may rarely metastasise to the walls of a larger bronchus. They may present identically to any primary proximal

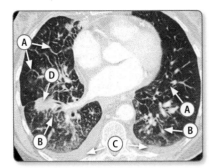

Figure 6.9 Computerised tomography scan showing lymphangitis. Ⓐ Thickened irregular interlobular septa, Ⓑ small nodules, Ⓒ small bilateral effusions, Ⓓ primary lung cancer.

tumour. The tumours are usually not evident on chest X-ray but may appear on CT scans. They can cause obstructive atelectasis of a lobe or lung. Bronchoscopic examination confirms the diagnosis if a tumour is suspected clinically.

Pleural disease

Most pleural disease presents with a pleural effusion, and affects 3000 people per million annually. Pleural effusions are a common symptom associated with more than 60 different diseases. **Table 7.1** lists the most likely causes.

Undiagnosed unilateral pleural effusions account for up to 5% of unselected medical admissions. Initial management usually involves pleural fluid sampling under ultrasound guidance to help narrow the wide range of differential diagnoses and relieve symptoms.

Occasionally, pleural disease presents with pleural thickening only. Pleural thickening restricts lung function, causing symptoms of breathlessness.

7.1 Mesothelioma and other pleural malignancies

Mesothelioma is an aggressive tumour that usually arises from the serosal surfaces of the pleura. It is expected to cause more than a quarter of a million deaths in Western Europe over the next 20 years. Almost all will result from previous asbestos

Type	Cause
Unilateral	Malignancy
	Pleural infection
	Cardiac failure
Bilateral	Cardiac failure
	Renal failure
	Liver failure

Table 7.1 The commonest causes of pleural effusions.

exposure. Inhaled asbestos fibres translocate from the lung to the pleura, where they damage pleural mesothelial cells. The period between asbestos exposure and the development of clinical symptoms is long, ranging between 15 and 60 years.

Clinical insight

Always consider mesothelioma in the differential diagnosis when a chest X-ray shows both a unilateral effusion and pleural plaques (**Figure 7.1**).

Clinical features

Patients tend to present with breathlessness caused by the pleural effusion. Over 90% of patients develop a pleural effusion during their illness. However, a small proportion develop pleural thickening only. Other common symptoms include:

- chest pain, often a localised dull ache over the chest wall
- weight loss and fatigue

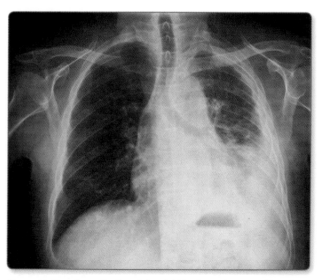

Figure 7.1 Chest X-ray of unilateral pleural thickening and associated loss of volume of the left hemithorax.

- sweating, which can be severe and results from release of cytokines from the mesothelioma.

Radiographic findings

Chest X-rays may show unilateral pleural effusion, pleural mass, pleural thickening and local rib invasion. Pleural plaques are also often present in cases of mesothelioma because of prior asbestos exposure.

7.2 Solitary fibrous tumour of the pleura

Solitary fibrous tumours of the pleura are benign pleural fibromas. They are uncommon and usually pedunculated.

Key facts

- Symptoms at presentation include cough, chest pain and dyspnoea.
- The tumours can grow extremely large before symptoms develop .
- Immunohistochemistry is extremely useful because solitary fibrous tumours of the pleura are vimentin-positive and keratin-negative with positivity for CD34.
- The tumours are usually benign but a small proportion can undergo malignant change.

Radiographic findings

Solitary fibrous tumours of the pleura appear as smooth, rounded, homogeneous masses on chest X-rays and usually occupy the lower zones (**Figures 7.2** and **7.3**). They have sharply delineated contours that form an obtuse angle with the pleural surface.

Management

Surgical excision (**Figure 7.4**) is the management of choice. Careful follow-up is needed because the tumours can recur. A small proportion undergo malignant change.

> ### Clinical insight
>
> In 1–2% of patients, solitary fibrous tumours of the pleura secrete insulin-like growth factor 2, which causes refractory hypoglycaemia. The condition usually resolves when the tumour is resected.

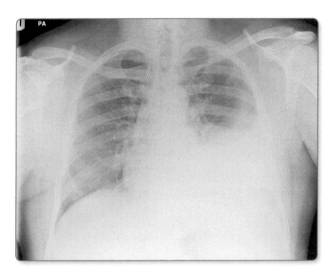

Figure 7.2 Chest X-ray showing a solitary fibrous tumour of the pleura.

7.3 Pleural infection

Pleural effusions occur in up to 40% of patients with pneumonia. Pleural infection affects patients of all ages but is more common in children and the elderly. Twice as many men are affected as women.

Parapneumonic effusions are the most common cause of pleural infection. Other causes include abdominal infection and intravenous drug or iatrogenic (e.g. after surgery).

Always consider parapneumonic collection when fever, pulmonary infiltrates and pleural fluid are present.

Clinical insight

Thoracic ultrasound is invaluable in the setting of pleural disease. Ultrasound identifies the extent of loculation and locates the best site for sampling pleural fluid and inserting a chest tube.

Radiographic findings

Consolidation and a simple pleural effusion are often

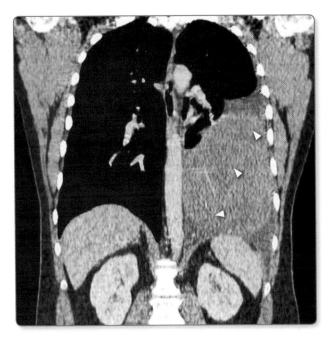

Figure 7.3 Computerised tomography scan of the thorax, showing a solitary fibrous tumour of the pleura (**arrowheads**).

seen and are usually unilateral. A D-shaped subpleural opacity is visible if pleural fluid has loculated (**Figure 7.5**). Inexperienced observers may misinterpret this finding as a lung mass. The presence of loculation or a low pleural fluid pH (<7.2) indicates the need for formal chest tube drainage in cases of pleural infection.

7.4 Pneumothorax

Pneumothorax is primary (in a normal underlying lung) or secondary (associated with underlying lung disease, e.g. chronic obstructive pulmonary disease, interstitial lung disease and cystic fibrosis). The annual incidence for primary and secondary pneumothorax is 24 in 100,000 men and 6 in 100,000 women.

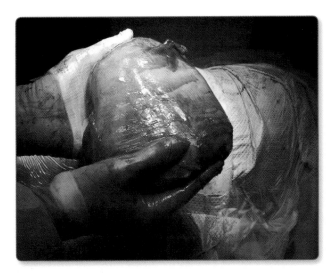

Figure 7.4 Solitary fibrous tumour of the pleura at the time of resection. By courtesy of Mr T Bachelor, Bristol, UK.

Pneumothoraces can also be iatrogenic (e.g. secondary to needle biopsy) or traumatic (e.g. after a fall with associated rib fractures). A tension pneumothorax occurs when air continues to enter the pleural cavity and cannot escape. This condition is potentially life-threatening.

Radiographic findings

Standard erect chest X-rays in inspiration are recommended for the initial diagnosis of pneumothorax. Expiratory films were previously advocated but are no longer thought to confer additional benefit in the routine assessment of pneumothorax.

Exercise diagnostic caution when using digital imaging (picture archiving and communication systems) to evaluate for pneumothorax. This is especially true when viewing on a desktop console with probably suboptimal screen size and pixel count on a brightly lit ward. Digital images are not ideal for

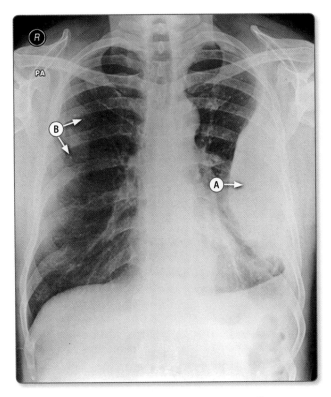

Figure 7.5 Chest X-ray showing a D-shaped subpleural opacity Ⓐ that needed chest tube drainage. Also present is miliary calcification caused by previous chickenpox pneumonitis Ⓑ.

measurement and size calculations. The auxiliary function of a cursor needs to be used to calculate the size of a pneumothorax. (Section 3.4 explains how to calculate pneumothorax size.)

Always look on a plain chest X-ray for the edge of the lung. The lung edge is normally absent but is visible in a pneumothorax (**Figure 7.6a**). X-rays are useful after drainage to document improvement (**Figure 7.6b**).

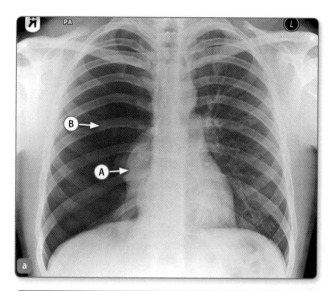

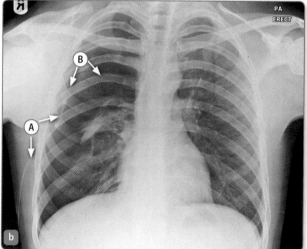

Figure 7.6 (a) Chest X-ray showing a complete right-sided spontaneous pneumothorax with atelectatic lung Ⓐ. Lung markings are absent from the right Ⓑ. (b) Chest X-ray after chest tube insertion Ⓐ. Partially reinflated lung Ⓑ.

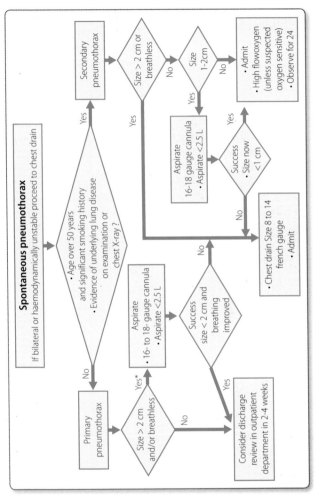

Figure 7.7 Algorithm from the 2010 British Thoracic Society guidelines on how to manage a pneumothorax. *Conservative management may be appropriate for some patients with a large pneumothorax but minimal symptoms. With permission from MacDuff A, Arnold A, Harvey J; BTS Pleural Disease Guideline Group. Management of spontaneous pneumothorax. British Thoracic Society pleural disease guideline 2010. Thorax 2010; 65 (Suppl 2): ii18–ii31.

Clinical insight

A computerised tomography scan of the thorax can help differentiate a pneumothorax from a bulla in a patient with chronic obstructive pulmonary disease. Placing a chest tube in a bulla by mistake can be life-threatening.

Management

The 2010 British Thoracic Society guidelines for pleural disease have a single algorithm for treatment of both primary and secondary pneumothorax (**Figure 7.7**). The algorithm is also available on the British Thoracic Society's website. Physicians should strongly emphasise to patients the need to stop smoking to minimise the risk of recurrence.

Secondary spontaneous pneumothorax is associated with higher morbidity and mortality than primary spontaneous pneumothorax. Therefore patients with secondary spontaneous pneumothorax should always initially receive in-patient care.

Mediastinal disease

This chapter covers a range of pathological conditions and abnormalities of the mediastinum, including the heart and great vessels. Section 3.5 covers evaluation of mediastinal masses and their differential diagnoses; however, a few examples are included here.

The chest X-ray frequently gives the first indication of pathological changes in the mediastinum and can sometimes allow a confident diagnosis to be made. At other times, the X-ray indicates the need for more detailed information from supplemental imaging tests, e.g. computerised tomography (CT), magnetic resonance imaging (MRI) and echocardiography.

8.1 Thymoma

Thymoma is a neoplasm of thymic epithelial cells (**Figure 8.1**) and accounts for 20–25% of mediastinal tumours. Mean age at presentation is 52 years. Serious complications occur because of compression of cardiopulmonary vessels and mediastinal structures.

Key facts
- Thymomas affect both sexes with equal frequency. They may be identified in 30–40% of patients with myasthenia gravis and are also associated with red cell aplasia and acquired hypogammaglobulinaemia.
- A spectrum of disease exists, with six histological and prognostic types (World Health Organisation classification). Thymic carcinoma has the worst prognosis.

Radiographic findings
Chest X-ray is non-specific and shows an anterior mediastinal mass. The differential diagnosis is therefore thymoma, teratoma, (terrible) lymph nodes and thyroid – the so-called

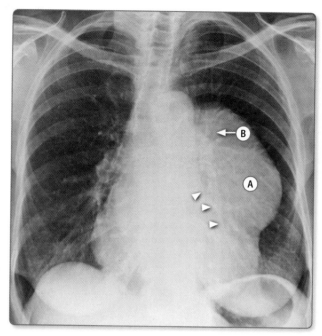

Figure 8.1 Chest X-ray showing a large mass with a smooth lobulated lateral margin (A). The medial border (arrowheads) abuts and silhouettes the left cardiac border, indicating that it is an anterior mediastinal mass. (B) Hilum overlay sign.

terrible Ts. Look for mass, loss of cardiac contour, the hilum overlay sign and visibility of posterior structures (e.g. the descending aorta). CT (**Figure 8.2**) allows more accurate anatomical localisation and refines the differential diagnosis. Positron emission tomography may predict malignancy. Resection is ultimately diagnostic.

Clinical insight

Normal thymus cannot be seen on chest X-ray in an adult but may be visible on CT–MRI, especially in patients younger than 30 years.

Management

Percutaneous biopsy of thymic tumours is safe and recommended prior to resection.

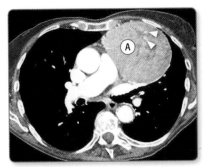

Figure 8.2 Axial computerised tomography scan at the level of the right main pulmonary artery. The mass (A) is of soft tissue density (similar to muscle) with peripheral vascularity (arrowheads).

8.2 Hiatus hernia

Hiatus hernia is a prolapsed portion of the stomach ascending into the thoracic cavity through the oesophageal hiatus (**Figure 8.3a**). It is categorised as sliding (prolapse of the portion of the stomach immediately inferior to the gastro-oesophageal junction) or rolling (prolapse of the fundus of the stomach).

Key facts
- Hiatus hernia is reportedly present in 70% of patients over 70 years old.
- Size varies greatly. Most hiatus hernias are asymptomatic and discovered incidentally. Rolling hiatus hernias tend to enlarge over time. Large hernias may become incarcerated, which may lead to strangulation or perforation.
- Sliding hernias predispose patients to oesophageal reflux, which over time may lead to oesophagitis and Barrett's oesophagus (cellular metaplasia).

Radiographic findings
In a hollow viscus, fluid will be dependent and form a sharp interface with air or an air–fluid level. An air–fluid level in a retrocardiac opacity is pathognomonic of hiatus hernia (**Figure 8.3b**). A lateral view may be useful if an air–fluid level is not visible; a barium swallow is an alternative sensitive

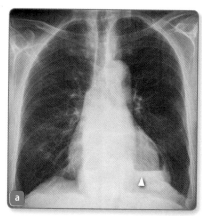

Figure 8.3 (a) Posteroanterior chest X-ray showing a retrocardiac opacity with an air–fluid level (arrowhead), typical of a large hiatus hernia. (b) Lateral view showing the hiatus hernia in the middle mediastinum. The wall of the stomach (A) is visible, with an air–fluid level (B) lying in the gastric lumen.

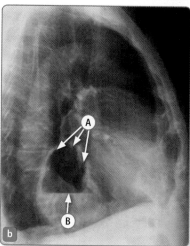

diagnostic test. If the patient has symptoms, endoscopy allows diagnosis as well as assessment of mucosal changes.

Management

Medical management relieves the symptoms of reflux and acid production. A larger hernia may require surgery (typically

Nissen fundoplication) to prevent volvulus (twisting) and potentially catastrophic infarction of the stomach.

8.3 Bronchogenic cyst

Bronchogenic cysts (**Figure 8.4**) are uncommon developmental anomalies resulting in an abnormal fluid-filled pouch lined with respiratory epithelium in the middle mediastinum or hilar region. They form part of a spectrum of abnormality classified as foregut duplication cysts.

Key facts
- Most patients present in the first few decades of life.
- Bronchogenic cysts may be asymptomatic or present with chest pain, cough or fever.

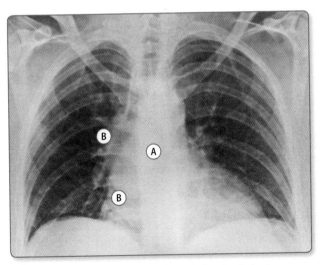

Figure 8.4 Chest X-ray showing a smooth mass in the subcarinal region: typically difficult to see. The carina is splayed Ⓐ, and an abnormal contour projects behind the heart to the right of the middle line and forms a convexity over the right main bronchus Ⓑ.

- The cysts may rarely cause dysphagia resulting from oesophageal compression.
- Sudden enlargement may be the result of internal haemorrhage, infection or distension with air.

Radiographic findings

A bronchogenic cyst is visible as a well-circumscribed hilar or middle mediastinal mass. Its appearance is non-specific and on chest X-ray raises a differential diagnosis of lymph node enlargement or oesophageal masses. An air–fluid level may be seen in infection and may mimic hiatus hernia.

Further imaging confirms location and can help characterise the cyst. Most cysts are of fluid density on CT (**Figure 8.5**), but the fluid is occasionally proteinaceous and may be of soft

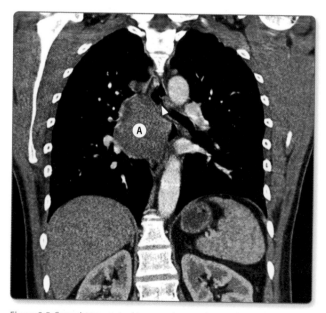

Figure 8.5 Coronal computerised tomography scan of same patient as in Figure 8.4, showing a fluid density mass (A) arising in the subcarinal region (carina - arrowhead).

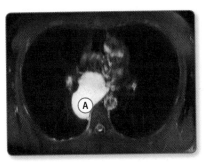

Figure 8.6 Axial T2-weighted magnetic resonance imaging scan showing the abnormality (A) in the mediastinum as high signal, indicating that it is composed of fluid.

tissue density. Lack of compression of adjacent structures and moulding of the cyst itself help show its fluid nature.

Magnetic resonance imaging (**Figure 8.6**) can provide supportive evidence with clear tissue characterisation. Simple fluid cysts are low signal on T1-weighted sequences but are bright T2-weighted images. Proteinaceous fluid is bright on both T1-weighted and T2-weighted sequences.

Management

Most cysts are removed surgically to either manage symptoms or prevent complications.

8.4 Retrosternal goitre

A retrosternal goitre (**Figure 8.7**) is an abnormally enlarged thyroid gland extending behind the sternum. Abnormal growth may cause various compressive syndromes because the thyroid gland is close to the trachea, larynx, superior and inferior laryngeal nerves, and oesophagus.

Key facts

- Goitres are common (present in up to 15% of the UK population).
- The commonest cause worldwide is iodine insufficiency.
- Patients with a goitre may have increased, normal or decreased thyroid function.

Radiographic findings

Retrosternal goitres appear on X-ray as superior mediastinal masses that can be localised to the anterior mediastinum. The mass appears to fade as it passes above the clavicle, indicating that the lesion extends from the neck anteriorly. Masses may be unilateral and shift the trachea away from the lesion, or they may be bilateral (**Figure 8.7**).

Thoracic inlet X-rays were historically used to evaluate tracheal compression resulting from a retrosternal goitre. CT is now preferred and accurately assesses the trachea and the anatomy of the goitre (**Figure 8.8**). Ultrasound is of limited use in assessing retrosternal extension because the beam cannot pass through bone. However, it can be used to confirm the impression of a goitre.

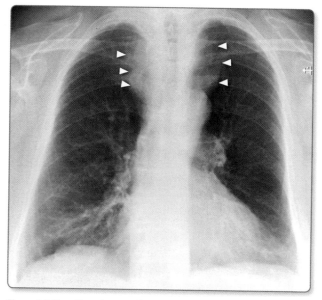

Figure 8.7 Chest X-ray showing a large goitre with bilateral retrosternal extension, visible as opacification in the superior mediastinum fading as it extends above the clavicles (arrowheads).

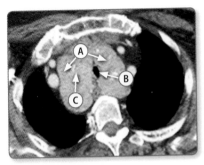

Figure 8.8 Axial computerised tomography scan at the level of the thoracic inlet, showing retrosternal extension of both lobes of the thyroid (A). This results in soft tissue encircling the trachea (B), which is narrowed by up to half of its normal diameter. Coarse calcification (C) in the thyroid tissue is a feature of benign disease (cf. microcalcification).

Management

Medical therapy is used for non-compressive, benign goitres. Treatment of hypothyroidism or hyperthyroidism often reduces the size of a goitre. The size of a benign euthyroid goitre may be reduced with levothyroxine suppressive therapy. Surgery is appropriate for large goitres with compression, malignant thyroid disease and goitres that fail to respond to other forms of therapy.

> **Clinical insight**
>
> Retrosternal goitres are common. Discovery on chest X-ray should prompt confirmatory ultrasound and potentially thyroid function testing.

8.5 Pneumomediastinum

The presence of gas in the mediastinum (**Figure 8.9**) indicates perforation of either the respiratory or the alimentary tracts. Gas-forming organisms may rarely be the source of non-anatomical gas arising from, for example, a retropharyngeal abscess or mediastinitis.

Key facts

- Symptoms of spontaneous pneumomediastinum include chest pain and dyspnoea.
- Spontaneous alveolar rupture is seen in young patients with a history of asthma or severe coughing or vomiting.

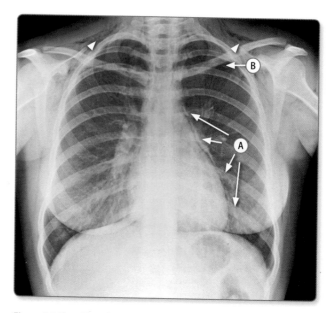

Figure 8.9 Chest X-ray showing pneumomediastinum and pneumothorax. Gas contours the mediastinum on the left Ⓐ. Left pneumothorax Ⓑ is associated with subcutaneous emphysema (arrowheads).

Rupture may also result from mechanical ventilation in any age group. Alveolar rupture leads to dissection of air through the pulmonary interstitium into the mediastinum and sometimes also into the pleural space to produce a pneumothorax.

• Alimentary tract injury is most commonly iatrogenic and found in the context of endoscopy.

Radiographic findings

Pneumomediastinum appears as streaks; bubbles; or collections of gas outlining the mediastinum, major airways, oesophagus or diaphragm. Air may dissect extrapleurally under the parietal layer of the mediastinal pleura, producing a thick linear opacity paralleling the cardiac border. Alternatively, air may extend between the heart and diaphragm, giving rise to the continuous diaphragm sign.

Distinguishing pneumomediastinum from pneumopericardium may be difficult. Air confined to the pericardium is classically thought not to extend above the base of the aortic arch or into the superior mediastinum.

Management

Pneumomediastinum is generally treated conservatively; surgery is of little value. Mechanical ventilation is occasionally warranted in cases associated with severe respiratory compromise, despite its potential to induce further air leaks.

8.6 Mitral regurgitation

Mitral regurgitation (**Figure 8.10**) is caused by failure of complete closure of the mitral valve during ventricular systole, resulting in retrograde passage of oxygenated blood from the left ventricle into the left atrium.

Key facts

- Mitral incompetence has multiple causes, including myocardial infarction, senile degeneration, rheumatic heart disease and connective tissue disorders.
- In acute mitral regurgitation, the small left atrium cannot cope with the sudden volume overload. The resulting pressure is transmitted to the pulmonary veins, causing pulmonary oedema. Chronic mitral regurgitation causes dilatation of both the left atrium and the left ventricle. Resulting symptoms include dyspnoea, pulmonary oedema and fatigue.
- Echocardiography provides functional and morphological evaluation of the heart and valve.

Radiographic findings

Chronic findings are cardiomegaly (increased cardiothoracic ratio) with left ventricular hypertrophy (seen as lateral

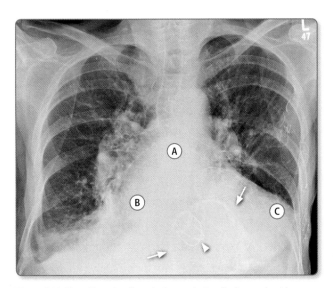

Figure 8.10 Chest X-ray showing mitral regurgitation. Cardiomegaly with enlargement of the left atrium (splaying of the carina (A) and 'second right heart border' (B)) and ventricle (C). A small right-sided pleural effusion is present. The mitral annulus calcification (arrowhead) is a common finding usually not associated with significant cardiac dysfunction. A metallic mitral valve prosthesis (arrows) and sternotomy wires are visible.

displacement of the left heart border) and left atrial dilatation. The left atrium is the most posterior aspect of the heart; dilatation results in an opacity medial to and paralleling the right side of the heart. Because of its location, the dilated left atrium may cause splaying of the carina and compression of the oesophagus (potentially causing dysphagia). Other findings include features of heart failure.

Management

Medical management involves the use of nitrates and antihypertensive drugs to reduce ventricular afterload. Mitral valve repair or replacement is indicated in chronic severe mitral regurgitation in patients who meet agreed criteria.

8.7 Pericardial effusion

The pericardial space normally contains 15–50 mL of fluid. Accumulation of excessive fluid (**Figure 8.11**) may result from local or systemic disorders and may be acute or chronic. Rapid accumulation of even a small volume of excess fluid may cause significant haemodynamic compromise, whereas

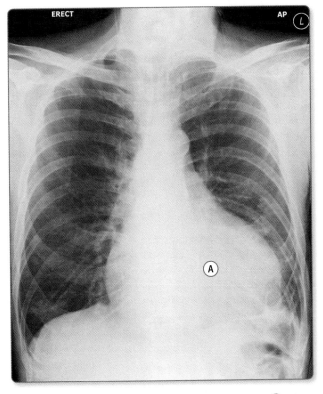

Figure 8.11 Chest X-ray showing pericardial effusion: enlarged heart Ⓐ with unusual globular shape.

chronic effusions may be as large as 2 L but be well compensated.

Key facts

- Over half of the occurrences of pericardial effusion are caused by a pre-existing condition (**Table 8.1**).
- Cardiac tamponade may result from rapidly accumulating fluid or very large effusions. However, small volumes of fluid or slow accumulation may be asymptomatic or result in limited signs.
- Echocardiography is the ideal imaging modality for detecting pericardial fluid, but it is also clearly visible on CT (**Figure 8.12**) and MRI.

> **Clinical insight**
>
> Classic clinical signs of tamponade are the Beck triad: hypotension, muffled heart sounds and increased jugular venous pressure. Tamponade may ultimately lead to cardiac arrest and causes pulseless electrical activity.

Radiographic findings

Typical findings are an enlarged cardiac outline caused by an increased cardiothoracic ratio, resulting in a characteristic globular shape (water bottle–shaped heart). A third of patients have a coexisting pleural effusion. Classic signs on X-ray are unfortunately uncommon. Consider the diagnosis in patients whose cardiac contour alters abruptly between films, but X-ray lacks sensitivity and specificity.

Cause	Examples
Idiopathic	
Infection	Coxsackievirus A and B are the commonest causes of infective pericarditis and myocarditis
Malignancy	Most commonly metastatic spread from bronchogenic malignancy
Postoperative	

Table 8.1 Common causes of pericardial effusions

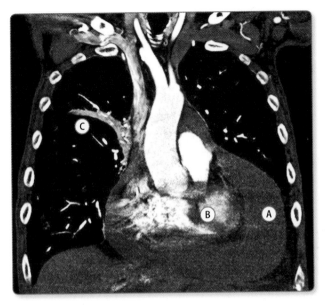

Figure 8.12 Coronal reconstruction from a computerised tomography scan of the same patient as in Figure 8.11. A large pericardial effusion (A) surrounds the heart (B). Some incidental linear atelectasis has developed in the right upper zone since the chest X-ray (C).

Management

Small effusions in haemodynamically stable patients are usually treated medically. Echocardiographically guided aspiration allows both treatment and diagnostic sampling of clinically significant effusions. Blind pericardiocentesis may be needed in resuscitation settings.

8.8 Aortic dissection

Dissection is caused by haemorrhage into the muscular layers of the aortic wall, resulting in a longitudinal split. Extension of the defect is common and may involve any branch of the thoracic or abdominal aorta. This may result in neurological complications and infarction of the abdominal viscera or even the lower limbs. Retrograde extension into the aortic root can cause haemopericardium or aortic insufficiency. Dissection is potentially life-threatening.

Key facts

- Presentation is usually acute, although untreated dissections may result in a chronic dissection flap that can be stable.
- Chest or back pain is the main symptom in 80–90% of cases. Examination classically shows a marked discrepancy between the blood pressure of each arm. Other signs may result from complications of extension, e.g. neurolwogical symptoms.
- All the multiple causes of aortic dissection result in medial necrosis, which leaves the muscle prone to tearing. The commonest cause is hypertension. Other causes include collagen disorders (e.g. Marfan syndrome) and congenital conditions (e.g. aortic coarctation).

Radiographic findings

The mediastinum is widened on chest X-ray; this effect is difficult to assess in supine and anteroposterior images. One highly specific sign is medial displacement of mural calcification resulting from blood tracking in the muscle layers of an abnormally dilated aortic arch (**Figure 8.13**). Additional signs (seen in Figure 8.13) that may be present include:

- a left apical cap visible as a crescent-shaped opacification in the left apex
- tracheal deviation
- pleural effusion.

The chest X-ray is normal in a quarter of patients but is recommended to rule out pneumothorax or pneumomediastinum, which mimic dissection. CT angiography is the first-line investigation if reasonable clinical suspicion exists. Echocardiography (transoesophageal) or MRI are alternative imaging modalities.

Clinical insight

Chest X-rays are a poor test for evaluating aortic dissection. CT or MRI is needed if clinical concern exists.

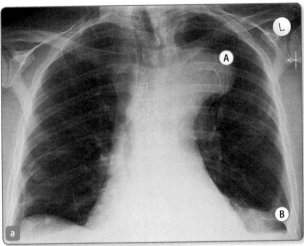

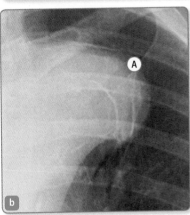

Figure 8.13 (a) Chest X-ray showing marked enlargement of the aortic knuckle. The mural calcification is medially displaced over the lateral aspect of the aortic arch (A) (B) Small associated left-sided pleural effusion. (b) Enlarged image of the aortic knuckle, clearly showing medial displacement of the mural calcification (A).

Management

Dissections are commonly subdivided using the Stanford classification into type A (involving the ascending aorta) or type B (limited to the descending aorta). Refer patients with type A dissections to a cardiothoracic surgical unit. Type B tears are generally managed medically by managing hypertension.

Airway pathology

This chapter describes the more common airway-related diseases except malignancy, which Chapter 6 covers.

9.1 Asthma

Asthma is an inflammatory abnormality of mainly medium-sized airways. The bronchi react abnormally to certain stimuli. Airflow is reversibly reduced and mucoid impaction may sometimes cause obstruction. The causes of asthma are complex and include both genetic and environmental factors. The disorder is common and its incidence increasing in most countries.

Radiographic findings

The chest X-ray in uncomplicated asthma is either normal or shows hyperinflated lungs (**Figure 9.1**). Subtle evidence of bronchial wall thickening may be present, more commonly in children.

A chest X-ray is indicated in acute asthma to exclude the following complications.

- Atelectasis caused by mucoid impaction of the airways.
- Consolidation caused by infection or acute allergic bronchopulmonary aspergillosis (ABPA).
- ABPA: proximal bronchiectasis and upper lobe fibrosis.
- Pneumomediastinum or pneumothorax.
- Churg–Strauss syndrome.

9.2 Allergic bronchopulmonary aspergillosis

Allergic bronchopulmonary aspergillosis is caused by the airways becoming hypersensitive to a species of the fungus *Aspergillus*. Virtually all patients have a history of asthma, atopy or both. The disease has a relapsing and remitting course. ABPA usually presents with asthma-like symptoms but systemic symptoms (e.g. fever, malaise and weight loss) are frequent.

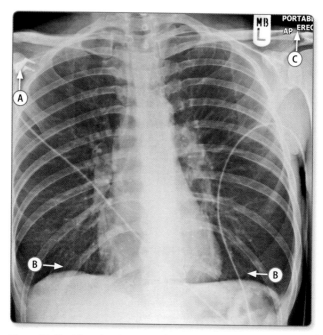

Figure 9.1 Chest X-ray showing acute asthma. The patient is sick – electrocardiogram leads are placed and it is a portable film. Ⓐ Electrocardiogram lead. Ⓑ Diaphragms depressed and flattened by hyperinflation. Ⓒ Anteroposterior portable labels.

Expectoration of large sputum plugs containing fungal mycelia is a helpful pointer to the diagnosis.

The diagnosis of ABPA can be difficult but is made from a combination of features including findings on X-ray (**Table 9.1**). It is important to distinguish ABPA from uncomplicated asthma because treatment for the two disorders differs.

Radiographic findings

The main feature on X-ray to suggest ABPA is a history of opacities. These may be multiple and vary from small nodules

Investigation	Results in allergic bronchopulmonary aspergillosis
Chest X-ray	History of flitting opacities
	Central bronchiectasis
	Varicose and cystic types
Blood tests	Blood eosinophilia
	Raised serum immunoglobulin E
Aspergillus-specific tests	Immediate skin reaction to *Aspergillus* antigen
	Precipitin antibodies to *Aspergillus* antigen

Table 9.1 Features used to diagnose allergic bronchopulmonary aspergillosis

to large segmental consolidations. Their cause is unclear; they are not true infections and may relate to airway obstruction or eosinophilic infiltrates. They may last for several weeks.

Computerised tomography (CT) may show the other features of ABPA, i.e. airway plugging and bronchiectasis. Areas of scarring and fibrosis may be visible in chronic disease and are usually predominantly in the upper zone. The changes become more apparent in chronic severe disease, as shown in the X-ray in **Figure 9.2**.

Clinical insight

Bronchiectasis is much less prevalent in uncomplicated asthma than in ABPA. Bronchiectasis is seen in chronic asthma but is usually more peripheral, milder and cylindrical.

9.3 Churg–Strauss syndrome

This chapter includes Churg–Strauss syndrome because it frequently presents with asthma symptoms and allergic rhinitis. The disorder is an uncommon autoimmune small-vessel vasculitis associated with perinuclear antineutrophil cytoplasm antibodies in about half of cases. It is important to recognise Churg–Strauss syndrome because it can progress to an extensive multiorgan disease if not treated early.

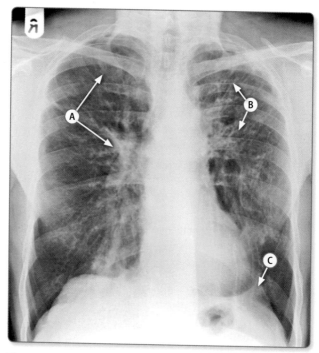

Figure 9.2 Chest X-ray showing chronic allergic bronchopulmonary aspergillosis. (A) Elevated hila and upper zone linear shadowing caused by fibrosis. (B) Upper zone tubular and ring shadows caused by bronchiectasis. (C) Tenting of the diaphragm, a sign of volume loss when the inferior pulmonary ligament pulls the diaphragm upwards.

Key facts

Clinical features of Churg–Strauss syndrome are:
- association with positive antineutrophilic cytoplasmic antibodies
- association with asthma (almost always present)
- marked peripheral eosinophilia
- paranasal sinusitis
- varying pulmonary consolidations

- small-vessel vasculitis on biopsy
- neuropathy.

Radiographic findings

The chest X-ray may be abnormal in up to about three quarters of patients in the earlier eosinophilic or vasculitic phases. The most common findings are pulmonary opacities, which may be nodular, mass-like or consolidative (**Figure 9.3**). The characteristic feature of Churg–Strauss syndrome is that the opacities vary in position and size over time. Features later in the disease process may be predominantly of a systemic vasculitis affecting many organs, particularly the heart, kidneys and gastrointestinal tract.

9.4 Chronic obstructive pulmonary disease

Chronic obstructive pulmonary disease is a spectrum of disorders but the term is most usually used to describe chronic bronchitis and emphysema. The two diseases commonly occur in the same patient. The two processes overlap clinically but one is often predominant in the radiographic findings, which are quite different. Most cases of chronic obstructive pulmonary disease are directly linked to long-term smoking.

Key facts

Chronic bronchitis is a clinical diagnosis characterised by a recurrent or chronic increase in production of bronchial secretions on most days for at least 3 months in two or more successive years. Pathological features involve airway mucous gland overactivity and inflammatory infiltrates. Airway obstruction is less reversible than in uncomplicated asthma.

Emphysema is a strictly pathological diagnosis. The characteristic finding is destruction of airspace walls and permanent enlargement of airspaces. Airways are obstructed because of loss of airway support from surrounding tissues and inflammation in small airway walls. The disease is classified based on the predominant area of the airspaces involved: centrilobular, paraseptal

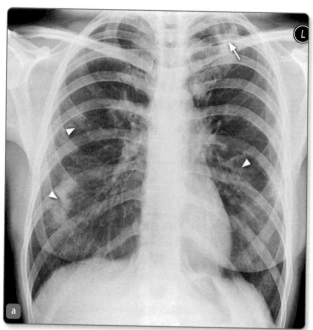

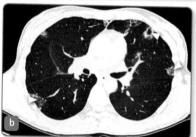

Figure 9.3 (a) Chest X-ray showing Churg–Strauss syndrome. Ill-defined areas of opacification in both lungs (arrowheads). (b) Computerised tomography scan from the same patient showing multiple areas of airspace opacification (arrowheads).

or panlobular. These areas can be assessed on high-resolution CT. The distinction is more difficult on X-rays when the emphysema is diffuse. Focal large bullae can become obvious when they develop. The predominant type of emphysema in smokers is centrilobular, which is usually most developed in the upper zones; these are the most obviously affected areas on X-rays.

Radiographic findings

Chronic bronchitis The chest X-ray is usually normal or shows hyperinflation (**Figure 9.4**). Subtle evidence of bronchial wall thickening may be present. The hyperinflation may be a sign of coexisting emphysema. Signs of pulmonary hypertension

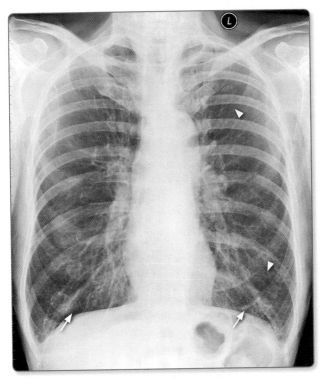

Figure 9.4 Chest X-ray showing chronic obstructive pulmonary disease. Diaphragms depressed and flattened by hyperinflation (arrows). Sparse coarse lung markings with bronchial wall thickening (arrowheads).

with enlargement of the proximal pulmonary vessels may be present in severe or advanced disease.

Emphysema The X-ray may appear normal in mild disease. The lungs are hyperinflated, as shown by low, flat diaphragms; increased retrosternal airspace; and narrow cardiac diameter.

Additional features are more subjective and relate to vascular changes. The lungs appear darker, i.e. more transradiant. Vessels are fewer and smaller; they are also distorted and straightened. Also visible are avascular spaces with hairline curvilinear margins caused by edges of focal bullae.

Emphysematous bullae are thin-walled, distended airspaces of >1 cm. They communicate with the airways but have no functional use and can expand to compress detrimentally adjacent normal lung (**Figure 9.5**). Emphysematous bullae may be multiple and can become large (>10 cm). They can cause complications such as pneumothorax, infection and haemorrhage. Bullae can also be mistaken clinically and radiographically for pneumothoraces.

Clinical insight

Beware of placing chest drains for a pneumothorax if it may be a large bulla. Obtain a CT scan of the patient if any doubt exists.

9.5 Alpha 1-antitrypsin deficiency

Alpha 1-antitrypsin is a serum peptide that inhibits proteases during inflammation. Lack of alpha 1-antitrypsin causes tissue damage from elastases released by macrophages and neutrophils. In the lungs, this results in emphysema. The deficiency is inherited. The clinical result is early onset of symptoms of chronic obstructive pulmonary disease.

Key facts

- Alpha 1-antitrypsin deficiency is one of the most common lethal inherited disorders.
- Homozygous persons eventually develop early-onset emphysema even if they are non-smokers.

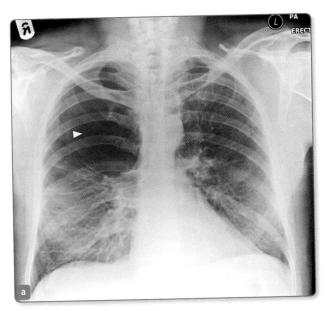

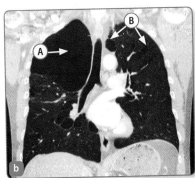

Figure 9.5 (a) Chest X-ray showing an emphysematous bulla. Large lucent area (arrowhead) with few lung markings and displacement or compression of adjacent lung and hilum. (b) Computerised tomography scan of emphysematous bulla. (A) Large right upper zone bulla. (B) Smaller areas of emphysema, both paraseptal and centrilobular in type.

- Heterozygous persons have varying degrees of milder disease, which is more severe if they smoke.
- It can also cause liver cirrhosis.

Radiographic findings

The emphysema is predominantly panacinar (panlobular). This is the most severe form. It affects all zones but an often striking lower zone predominance is present in alpha 1-antitrypsin deficiency (**Figure 9.6**). Bullous formation is rare and additional bronchiectasis may be present.

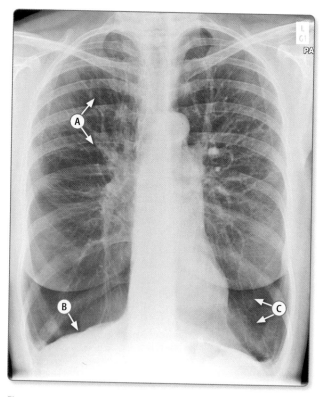

Figure 9.6 Chest X-ray showing alpha 1-antitrypsin deficiency. (A) Normal upper zone lung markings. (B) Diaphragms flattened by hyperinflation. (C) The lower zones have emphysema: more lucency with sparse lung markings.

9.6 Bronchiectasis and cystic fibrosis

Bronchiectasis and cystic fibrosis are discussed together because the basic abnormality on X-ray is bronchiectasis in both diseases.

Bronchiectasis is a chronic condition of irreversible bronchial dilatation caused by inflammation. It should be distinguished from the temporary dilatation frequently seen in pneumonia and atelectasis. There are many causes and associations (**Table 9.2**). Some examples are included elsewhere, such as ABPA and bronchiectasis as a result of fibrosis causing traction bronchial dilatation (e.g. after radiation, sarcoid and interstitial lung disease).

Cystic fibrosis is an autosomal recessive inherited condition that is relatively common in white populations but rare

Cause	Example(s)
Previous infection	Childhood infection
	Measles
	Tuberculosis
	Pertussis
Obstruction to airway with postobstructive dilatation	Tumour
	Foreign body
	Extrinsic compression of airway by lymph nodes
Impaired immune defences	Cystic fibrosis
	Immune deficiencies
Allergy	Allergic bronchopulmonary aspergillosis
Fibrosis	End-stage traction bronchial dilatation
Miscellaneous	Rheumatoid arthritis
	Congenital condition

Table 9.2 Common causes of bronchiectasis

in Asia and Africa. The disease involves abnormal production of mucosal and pancreatic secretions. The lungs are the most severely affected organ. Chronic inspissation of mucus, together with airway infection, eventually causes severe bronchiectasis, particularly in the mid and upper zones of lungs. Life expectancy has historically been poor but modern treatments allow more patients to reach adulthood.

Key facts

- Clinical symptoms, particularly in more severe disease, are chronic cough, copious purulent sputum production and repeated respiratory infections.
- Patients may present with haemoptysis.
- Cor pulmonale may develop in widespread progressive disease.

Radiographic findings

Bronchiectasis is now diagnosed by high-resolution CT. It was historically diagnosed using bronchography, a technique sometimes still used in children. The condition is classified into three types according to severity: cylindrical (milder), varicose (more dilated and irregular) and cystic (severe disease with large focal ballooning).

Only severe disease is usually apparent on plain chest X-rays. The dilated airways appear as tubular, parallel, linear opacities (**Figure 9.7**) or as ring shadows if seen end on. Consolidation may also be seen in acute infection.

Findings on high-resolution CT are essentially the same but milder disease is apparent. Airways are normally seen next to pulmonary arteries and the airway is smaller than the adjacent vessel. The walls of bronchiectatic airways are thickened and the lumen larger than the artery (**Figure 9.8**). There may also be plugging of small airways, which are usually not seen on CT; this causes a branching opacity termed tree in bud.

The extent of bronchiectasis depends on the cause. It may be localised to a small segment or be widespread, e.g. in cystic fibrosis.

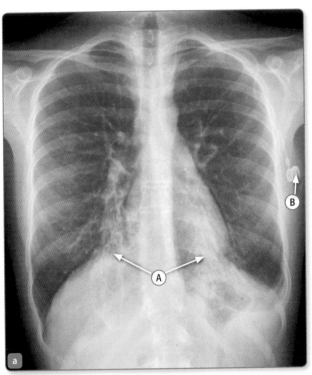

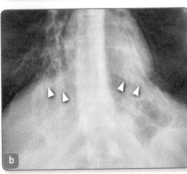

Figure 9.7 Chest X-ray showing bronchiectasis (a) **(A)** Crowding of lung markings with increased linear opacities. **(B)** Subcutaneous portocath placed for regular intravenous injections of antibiotics. (b) Magnified view showing parallel and tubular opacities caused by dilated bronchi (arrowheads).

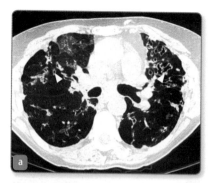

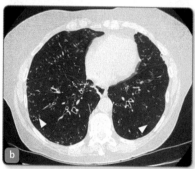

Figure 9.8 High-resolution computerised tomography appearance of bronchiectasis. (a) Thick-walled dilated airways (arrowheads). (b) Peripheral small branching opacities (arrowheads) caused by plugged terminal airways ('tree in bud' opacities) with distal air trapping.

Radiographic changes associated with cystic fibrosis may not develop for several years. The first signs may be bronchial wall thickening and hyperinflation. Progression eventually leads to changes mainly in the upper zones of extensive bronchiectasis (**Figure 9.9**) and complications such as atelectasis, consolidations and hilar adenopathy. Large bronchiectatic cavities may develop air–fluid levels. Pneumothorax and severe haemoptysis may occur.

9.7 Inhaled foreign body

Inhalation of foreign bodies is much more common in small children but also occurs more frequently in the elderly or

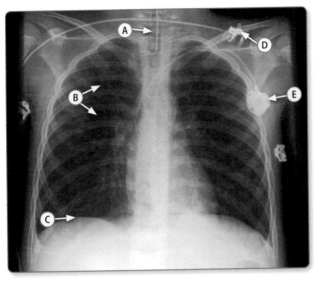

Figure 9.9 Chest X-ray showing cystic fibrosis. (A) Endotracheal tube. (B) Upper zone ring shadows and tubular opacities caused by bronchiectasis. (C) Diaphragms flattened by hyperinflation, although note that the patient is ventilated. (D) Electrocardiogram lead. (E) Portacath for regular intravenous antibiotic therapy.

very ill. The most common items are peanuts, other foods and broken teeth.

Radiographic findings

A dense object may be apparent on a chest X-ray. However, usually only the effects of an inhaled foreign body are apparent, most commonly air trapped in the affected lobe or lung. The area is expanded and more lucent (**Figure 9.10**). This effect of air-trapping occurs as air is able to pass the foreign body into the lung, but less able to be exhaled. The object may be more apparent on X-rays obtained in expiration; the more normal lung will shrink and become more dense whereas the abnormal areas stay hyperinflated and lucent. Alternatively, if the airway is completely obstructed, the lobe or lung may

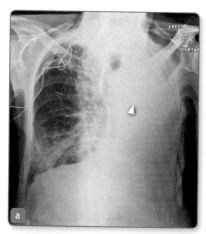

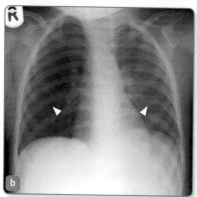

Figure 9.10 Chest X-ray showing inhaled foreign bodies. (a) Complete opacification of hemithorax (arrowhead) with shift to that side resulting from collapse of left lung from inhaled foreign body in the left main bronchus. (b)The right lung is hyperinflated and more lucent than the left (arrowheads) because of air trapped in the right main bronchus by an inhaled foreign body.

collapse completely (**Figure 9.10**). CT may also be helpful because it shows the same effects more clearly.

Management

Inhaled foreign bodies may cause pneumonia or atelectasis if not removed early. Bronchoscopy is necessary if an inhaled foreign body is suspected and will usually allow its removal.

Pulmonary oedema

Pulmonary oedema is accumulation of fluid in the lungs. It can lead to impaired gas exchange and ultimately respiratory failure. Its cause is either altered hydrostatic pressures or direct (acute) injury.

- Abnormal hydrostatic forces most commonly result from cardiac dysfunction and also occur in renal disease and fluid overload.
- Acute lung injury and acute respiratory distress syndrome (ARDS) causes fluid build-up by damaging capillary membranes and increasing their permeability.

10.1 Cardiogenic pulmonary oedema

Left cardiac dysfunction leads to increased pulmonary venous pressures and lymphatic drainage. Once the capacity of the pulmonary lymphatic vessels is exceeded, fluid seeps into the interstitium and then into the alveolar airspaces. This process may occur rapidly or gradually and may or may not occur in sequence. Assess cardiac size on posterior images; cardiomegaly indicates that oedema is probably cardiogenic.

Radiographic findings

Cardiac failure causes a spectrum of pulmonary findings: increased pulmonary venous pressure, interstitial oedema and alveolar oedema. The signs on X-ray depend on the severity of the increase in left atrial pressure.

Increased pulmonary venous pressure Cardiomegaly is commonly present (**Figure 10.1**). The vessels of the upper lobes are normally slightly smaller than lower lobe vessels on erect X-rays. An increased left atrial pressure of 16–22 cm of H_2O causes upper lobe blood diversion, which appears as dilation. Small effusions blunt the costophrenic angles.

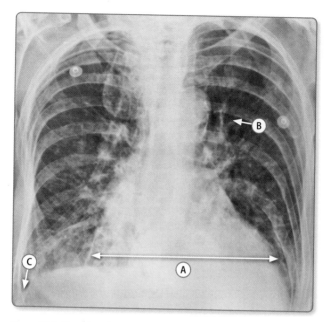

Figure 10.1 Chest X-ray showing interstitial oedema: cardiomegaly Ⓐ, upper lobe blood diversion Ⓑ, loss of clarity of perihilar vessels «B» and blunting of costophrenic recesses Ⓒ, indicating small effusions.

Interstitial oedema Interstitial oedema occurs at left atrial pressures of 22–30 cm of H_2O. The lung interstitium is an interconnecting connective tissue framework with central (perivascular, peribronchial) and peripheral (interlobular, subpleural) components. These elements thicken as fluid accumulates.

The following indicate interstitial thickening.

- Loss of clarity (hazing) of the perihilar vessels and thickening of the bronchial walls (peribronchial cuffing).
- Septal (or Kerley B) lines (**Figure 10.2**): peripheral, straight, short (1–2 cm), horizontal lines in contact with the parietal pleura in the lower zones.

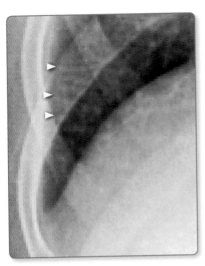

Figure 10.2 Close-up of chest X-ray showing right costophrenic recess with numerous Kerley B lines (arrowheads).

- Laminar effusions: a band of density against the lateral chest wall arising at the level of the costophrenic angle and resulting from subvisceral accumulation of pleural fluid.

Alveolar oedema Alveolar oedema (**Figure 10.3**) occurs when the left atrial pressure exceeds 30 cm of H_2O. Alveolar spaces become opacified (consolidated) by fluid. In pulmonary oedema this airspace opacification is usually bilateral and has a perihilar ('bat's wing') distribution in pulmonary oedema. Pulmonary oedema can develop and resolve quickly, which helps distinguish it from infection.

10.2 Acute lung injury and acute respiratory distress syndrome

Acute lung injury (**Figure 10.4**) is defined as acute respiratory symptoms with radiographic infiltrates but no evidence of left heart failure and a PaO_2 or FiO_2 >300 mmHg. Acute respiratory distress syndrome (ARDS) is defined as acute respiratory

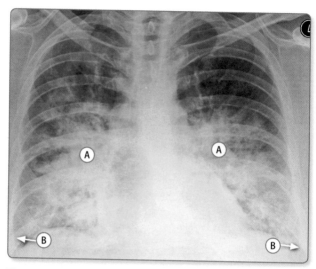

Figure 10.3 Chest X-ray showing alveolar oedema: airspace opacification in the perihilar regions (A) producing a bat's wing appearance. Both costophrenic recesses are blunted (B), indicating small effusions.

symptoms with radiographic infiltrates but no evidence of left heart failure and a PaO_2 or FiO_2 >200 mmHg.

Key facts

- Lung injury may be direct (primary) or indirect (secondary). Patients present with respiratory distress and appropriate history.
- Common primary causes are aspiration, pulmonary infection, near drowning, inhalation of toxic fumes and lung contusion.
- Common secondary causes are systemic sepsis, severe non-thoracic trauma, hypertransfusion and cardiopulmonary bypass.

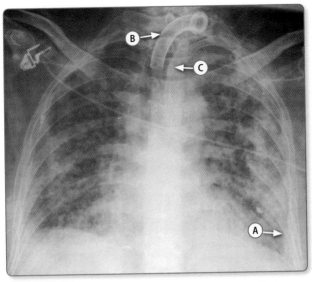

Figure 10.4 Chest X-ray showing the bilateral patchy airspace opacification typical of acute respiratory distress syndrome. Ⓐ Bilateral chest drains, Ⓑ tracheostomy, Ⓒ nasogastric tube.

Radiographic findings

The chest X-ray may be normal in the first 24 h of secondary ARDS. The first sign is widespread 'ground glass' opacification, which progresses to widespread airspace opacification over the next 36 h.

Bilateral airspace opacification is a non-specific finding, so ARDS may be indistinguishable from hydrostatic pulmonary oedema on X-ray. However, the appearance of ARDS on X-ray tends to plateau and persist for a variable time.

Positions of lines and tubes in the chest

The chest X-ray is essential for examining the positions of lines and tubes in the chest. Correct placement of a device and absence of complications must often be confirmed before the device can be used. Therefore knowledge of potential complications and correct positions is essential.

11.1 Nasogastric tubes

Follow local guidelines to ensure that the tube is correctly positioned (**Figure 11.1**) before feeding. Confirm correct position after insertion. An incorrectly placed nasogastric tube (**Figure 11.2**) carries a high risk of severe morbidity and mortality. Problems include:

- feeds delivered to the lungs (**Figure 11.2b**)
- pneumothorax (**Figure 11.3**)
- aspiration of feeds into the lungs if the tube is curled in the oesophagus or a hiatus hernia (**Figure 11.2a**).

Key facts

- Nasogastric tubes should be radiopaque or contain a metallic guide wire for the duration of the X-ray.
- An X-ray is indicated if the pH of aspirated fluid is outside the safe range of 1–5.5 (i.e. acidic because of gastric acid).
- The person responsible for checking the X-ray must be suitably qualified or, if not a radiologist, adequately trained.

Radiographic findings

Certain fundamental features should be assessed.

- Does the tube path follow the oesophagus and avoid the contours of the bronchi?
- Does the tube bisect the carina?
- Does it cross the diaphragm in the midline?
- Is the tip clearly below the diaphragm?

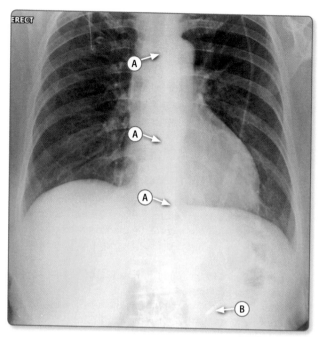

Figure 11.1 Chest X-ray showing the correct position for safe feeding through a nasogastric tube. (A) The line of the tube passes centrally and not through a main bronchus, staying close to the midline. (B) The tip of the tube is more dense and well below the diaphragm.

Feeding should start only if all the above criteria are satisfied. Seek advice from a more experienced practitioner if in any doubt.

11.2 Central venous lines and pacemakers

Venous access lines allow rapid administration of fluids or drugs through large vessels. They are essential if peripheral access is poor and large or rapid infusions are needed. Venous lines

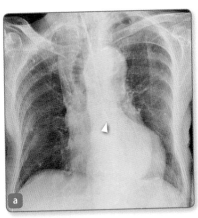

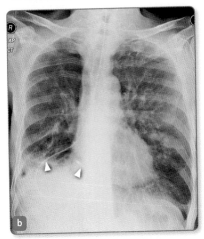

Figure 11.2 Chest X-rays showing incorrectly positioned nasogastric tubes. (a) The tip of the nasogastric tube (arrowhead) is curled in the lower oesophagus and is unsafe. (b) The nasogastric tube (arrowheads) passes into the right lung; the patient died after feed was delivered through this tube.

can also be used to monitor central pressures, helping to avoid excessive venous overload to the heart. Insertion is through a jugular or subclavian route.

Pacemaker wires are tunnelled under the skin and fed through the subclavian vein into the heart. The tip is in the wall

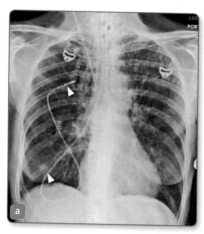

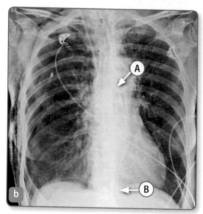

Figure 11.3 Chest X-rays showing incorrectly positioned nasogastric tubes. (a) A nasogastric tube (arrowheads) passes through the right main bronchus into the right lung, causing a subsequent tension pneumothorax. (b) A nasogastric tube (A) passes through the left main bronchus. (B) Although the tip of the tube appears to be below the diaphragm, it was in the posterior costophrenic recess and was unsafe for feeding.

of the right atrium, the right ventricle or both, as necessary, depending on the type of pacemaker. Complications of their insertion are similar to those of venous lines.

All central venous lines need to be placed in specific intravascular sites. A chest X-ray is useful to confirm that a line is correctly positioned, and that there are no complications.

- The tip of most central lines should be in the superior vena cava or brachiocephalic veins (**Figure 11.4a**).
- Dialysis catheters transmit large volumes and should be in the right atrium (**Figure 11.4b**).
- Pacemaker wires vary in their positioning; the tip of the wire should be documented at time of insertion rather than on subsequent X-ray.

Catheters are sometimes tunnelled through subcutaneous tissues to lessen the risk of infection if needed for prolonged periods. Large double-bore lines may be used for kidney dialysis.

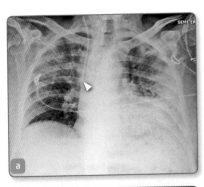

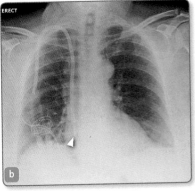

Figure 11.4 Chest X-rays showing right jugular lines. (a) Tip of the right jugular central venous line (arrowhead) projected over the lower superior vena cava. (b) Tip of a tunnelled right dialysis catheter (arrowhead) projected over the right atrium. No complications occurred in either case.

After insertion of any central venous access device, a chest X-ray is needed to check the position of the line and ensure that no complication has occurred. The most common potential complication is a pneumothorax (**Figure 11.5**). Injury to the vein or adjacent artery could cause bleeding into the pleural or extrapleural spaces or the mediastinum. Venous lines may pass retrogradely or into branch vessels, causing thrombosis, and should be repositioned (**Figure 11.6**).

11.3 Tracheal intubation

The trachea is intubated with an endotracheal tube or through a tracheostomy. The inferior tip of the tube should be about

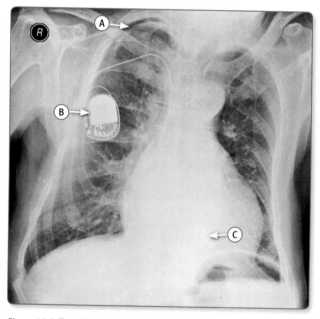

Figure 11.5 Chest X-ray showing a pneumothorax caused by insertion of a permanent pacemaker. (**A**) Apical pneumothorax. (**B**) Pacemaker box. (**C**) The tip of a pacemaker wire in the wall of the right ventricle.

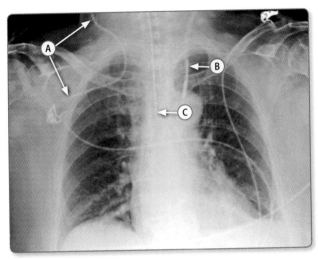

Figure 11.6 Chest X-ray showing a misplaced right jugular venous line. (A) The right jugular venous line passes from the jugular into the right subclavian vein and is unsafe. (B) The left jugular line passes into the left brachiocephalic vein. (C) The tip of the endotracheal tube is too low; it lies only just above the carina. The tube needs to be withdrawn by 2–3 cm.

2–3 cm above the carina. The opposite lung or an ipsilateral lobe may collapse if the tube is misplaced in a main bronchus. Anatomical variation needs to be considered during intubation. For example, in a patient in whom the tracheal origin of the right upper lobe airway is lower than usual, the airway can be obstructed by a tube placed at what would otherwise be the correct level (**Figure 11.7**).

11.4 Chest drains

Chest drains are used to drain pleural effusions and pneumo-thoraces, and can be left in place after thoracic surgery.

The tubes used in chest drains contain a radiopaque line to show their position. Towards the tip, as well as an end hole, they

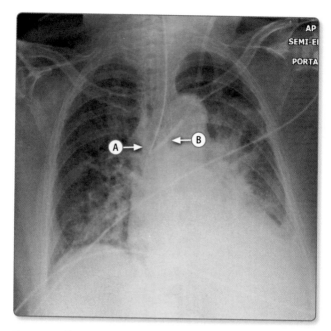

Figure 11.7 Chest X-rays showing misplaced endotracheal tubes. Ⓐ Tip of an endotracheal tube in the right main bronchus. The tube needs to be withdrawn into the correct position and the X-ray repeated. Ⓑ The left jugular venous line tip is in the left brachiocephalic vein, close to the superior vena cava.

have one or more side holes visible as gaps in the radiopaque line. It is important to ensure that the side holes are in the pleural space. Subcutaneous emphysema may develop if the side holes are extrapleural.

The tube may need to be manoeuvred into the affected area if effusions are loculated or a pneumothorax localised. Use posteroanterior views (**Figures 11.8 and 11.9**) to assess the position and monitor the effectiveness of treatment. Lateral or decubitus films sometimes also help.

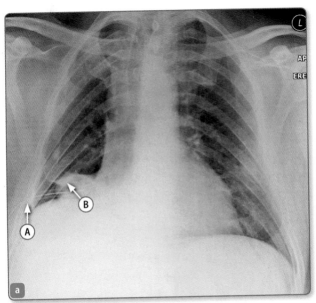

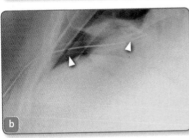

Figure 11.8 (a) Chest X-ray showing chest drain (A) entering the chest wall. Partially collapsed lobe not yet expanded (B) (so-called trapped lung). (b) Magnified view showing side holes in the drain tubing (arrowheads) lying in the chest.

11.5 Other devices and the intensive care situation

Take care to assess the multiple medical devices and leads on the skin that patients, particularly those who are ventilated,

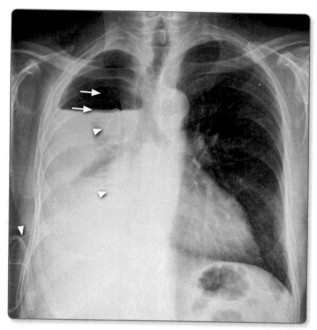

Figure 11.9 Chest X-ray showing chest drain in a large hydropneumothorax. Air–fluid level caused by air above the pleural fluid (arrows). Chest drain lying within the pleural collection (arrowheads).

may have. X-rays are frequently done in intensive care units just to monitor the positions of devices, lines and tubes and to ensure that no iatrogenic complications occur (**Figure 11.10**).

Other lines and devices to be aware of include abdominal drains, which may be misplaced or migrate through the diaphragm. Nephrostomy tubes (**Figure 11.10**) to drain obstructed kidneys may pass through the pleura and cause a pneumothorax or leak fluid above the diaphragm. Misplaced subphrenic or liver drains for draining abscesses may cause similar intrathoracic complications.

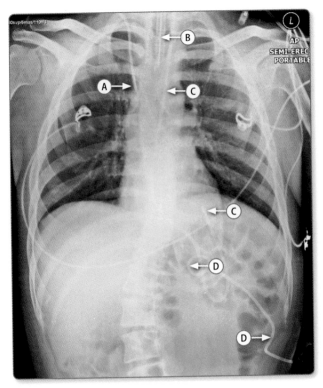

Figure 11.10 Chest X-ray showing multiple lines and tubes. Ⓐ Tip of the right jugular line projected over the superior vena cava. Ⓑ Endotracheal tube. Ⓒ Correctly placed nasogastric tube. Ⓓ Nephrostomy tube draining an obstructed left kidney.

Surgical changes are discussed elsewhere (see section 2.5). Various medical devices may be seen in the chest, e.g. the oesophageal stent and ventriculoperitoneal shunt in **Figure 11.11**. Superior vena cava and tracheobronchial stents have a metallic mesh and resemble oesophageal stents.

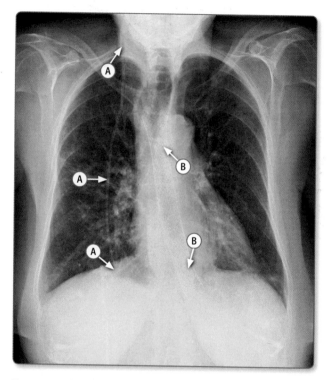

Figure 11.11 Chest X-ray showing other devices in the chest. **(A)** Ventriculoperitoneal shunt tube passing from the brain to the peritoneal cavity to drain obstructive hydrocephalus. **(B)** Long oesophageal stent to treat obstruction.

Index

Note: Page numbers in **bold** or *italic* refer to tables or figures respectively.